Praise for Kris Wilder...

Many practitioners believe that Sanchin Kata holds
al martial arts. It is one of the simplest forms to learn
most difficult to perfect. Those who truly understand
tates enormous quickness and power in any martial application. The challenge comes
in gaining that understanding, something we had to uncover by trial and error until
now. In his groundbreaking book, *The Way of Sanchin Kata*, Sensei Wilder lays out
step-by-step instructions for mastering this vital form. He covers every element of body
mechanics, movement, breathing, and application with clear writing, pertinent detail,
and informative illustrations. The "test it" exercises help readers internalize what they
have learned. Wilder manages to take the ancient wisdom of sanchin kata and make it
relevant for modern budoka today. If you want to develop real strength, speed,
endurance, and power for tournament competition or street survival you need to buy
this book. It should be required reading for any serious martial artist.

—**Lawrence A. Kane,** martial arts instructor; author of *Surviving
Armed Assaults* and co-author of *The Way of Kata*

I have heard (and failed to understand) that Sanchin is the core kata of Goju-ryu
Karate for 26 years. Mr. Wilder's book has finally shed light on why Sanchin is important. It has given me solid direction and guidance in pursuing Sanchin training for
myself. After 26 years in Goju, I am finally excited to study and practice this kata.

—**Dr. Jeff Cooper, M.D.,** Tactical Medical Director of
the Toledo Ohio SWAT; Commander, US Naval
Reserve; 4th degree black belt in Goju Ryu karate.

Sanchin is one of the most important karate kata. Unfortunately it is also one of
the most misunderstood. This great book by Kris Wilder dispels the myths surrounding Sanchin and explains all aspects of the kata in a straightforward and accessible way.
This thoughtful and intelligent book also reveals how to put the lessons of Sanchin to
the test so you can experience their effects firsthand. *The Way of Sanchin Kata* is a truly
great piece of work that all martial artists should read.

—**Iain Abernethy,** 5th Dan Karate (British Combat Association and
Karate England) and author of *Bunkai-Jutsu:
The Practical Application of Karate Kate*

This book has been sorely needed for generations! Mr. Wilder finally reveals the
sssence of Sanchin, the kata that is the cornerstone of Okinawan karate. This is truly a
fascinating book that explains more than just the "how," but also the "why." Moreover,
the concepts and principles presented in this text can be readily applied to many other
kata. Congratulations to Mr. Wilder on a masterful work that every serious karateka
absolutely must own!

—**Philip Starr,** *Inside Kung Fu* Hall of Fame Member; Founder of Yiliquan

The Way of
Sanchin Kata

残心

The Way of Sanchin Kata

The Application of Power

KRIS WILDER

YMAA Publication Center
Boston, Mass. USA

YMAA Publication Center, Inc.
Main Office:
 PO Box 480
 Wolfeboro, New Hampshire, 03894
 1-800-669-8892 • www.ymaa.com • ymaa@aol.com

Editor: Susan Bullowa
Cover Design: Richard Rossiter
Illustrated by Kris Wilder

ISBN-13: 978-1-59439-084-5
ISBN-10: 1-59439-084-3

POD0410

Publisher's Cataloging in Publication
Wilder, Kris A.

  The way of sanchin kata : the application of power / Kris Wilder. --
1st ed. -- Boston, Mass. : YMAA Publication Center, 2007.

    p. ; cm.

    ISBN-13: 978-1-59439-084-5
    ISBN-10: 1-59439-084-3
    Includes glossary, bibliographical references and index.

    1. Martial arts. 2. Karate. 3. Martial arts--Psychological aspects.
  4. Hand-to-hand fighting, Oriental. I. Title.

    GV1114.3 .W55 2007
    796.815/3--dc22   0704

Warning: Studying these materials may give you, or cause you to acquire, a certain degree of power that you did not previously possess. The authors and publisher expect you to use that power responsibly. Readers are encouraged to be aware of all appropriate local and national laws relating to self-defense, reasonable force, and the use of martial techniques in conflict situations and act in accordance with all applicable laws at all times. Neither the authors nor the publisher assume any responsibility for the use or misuse of information contained in this book.

All martial arts are, by their very definition, warlike and dangerous. Training should always be undertaken responsibly, ensuring every available precaution for the safety of all participants. No text, no matter how well written, can substitute for professional hands-on instruction. Consequently these materials should be used *for academic study only*.

Printed in USA.

Table of Contents

Acknowledgements. vii

Dedication ix

Foreword by Hiroo Ito xi

Thoughts on Hiroo Ito's Words xv

Preface xvii

Introduction xix

Chapter One: The History of Sanchin Kata 1

Chapter Two: Learning by Emulation and Repetition 5

Chapter Three: The Mechanics of Being in the Moment 7

Chapter Four: Measurement, Personal and Unique 15

Chapter Five: The Roots of a Strong Tree, the Feet 21

Chapter Six: Thighs 31

Chapter Seven: Hips 33

Chapter Eight: The Trunk of a Strong Tree 35

Chapter Nine: Movement Not Seen. 37

Chapter Ten: Crescent Step 43

Chapter Eleven: The Spine. 49

Chapter Twelve: Shoulders. 57

Chapter Thirteen: Arms. 59

Chapter Fourteen: The Fist 61

Chapter Fifteen: Knuckles 67

Chapter Sixteen: The Striking Arm 69

Chapter Seventeen: The Back. 79

Chapter Eighteen: The Energetic and Mechanical Structure. 83

Chapter Nineteen: The Iron Shirt 91

Chapter Twenty: Rooting. 99

Chapter Twenty-One: The Mind 103

Chapter Twenty-Two: Ten-Minute Sanchin Kata 107

Chapter Twenty-Three: Implements for Sanchin Kata Training 125

Chapter Twenty-Four: Breathing 139

Chapter Twenty-Five: Turning 143

Chapter Twenty-Six: The Kata 147

Conclusion 167

Notes. 169

Glossary. 173

Bibliography 177

Index 179

About the Author. 183

Acknowledgements

If you have knowledge, let others light their candles in it.

—*Margaret Fuller* [1]

Many teachers and associates have given freely of themselves asking little or nothing in return making this book possible. Without the selfless giving of the following people, this book would simply not be possible. Whether teacher, friend, student, or in some other role, each has contributed in their own ways. An immeasurable amount of appreciation goes to Hiroo Ito, a *karate-ka*, *sensei*, and seeker. It is simply impossible to thank him enough for his teaching, knowledge, and friendship. To Laura Vanderpool, for her reviewing of this book and bringing focus to the words, a brief sentence hardly describes the effort and her help. To Lawrence Kane, a friend, and fellow *karate-ka* who is always willing to give valuable encouragement and even more valuable criticism. Moreover, to the students who have, through their diligence, shown me more about myself and the art than I could have possibly learned otherwise.

Dedication

To my family who, with out exception, has always been a strong keel in storm or calm.

Foreword
by Hiroo Ito

Historic Background of Okinawa-Style Karate　那覇手系の型の流れ

昔から基本型（三戦）があり、その他応用技のための（砕破　サイファー）、
（制引戦　セイエンチン）、（四向戦　シソウチン）、（三十六手
サンセイリュウ　）（十八手　セイパイ）（久留頓破
クルルンファ）、（壱百零八手
スーパールンペ）が残っている。そして剛柔流に引き継がれ宮城長順が考案した
（撃砕第　ゲキサイ）　開手型の（転掌　テンショウ）等がある。
この中の基本型である三戦は基本、鍛錬型として、いかなる人でも‘この型に先
んじて他の型を演じてずることは許されない’と言うことが歴史の中で不文律と
して残っている。

The basic *kata sanchin* has existed a long time, and has developed into variations called *saifa, seiyunchin, shisochin, sanseiryu, seipai, kururunfa,* and *suparunpen,* which are still practiced. The *Goju-Ryu* karate formed by Chojun Miyagi created the *tensho kata,* which is an open-fisted *kata,* as opposed to the *gekisai kata.*

Sanchin is the basic *kata* used to build karate strength (*kanren kata*), which is the foundation for all of these *kata.* It has been an accepted historical fact that, "It is not possible to do any other *kata* without first having mastered the basic *sanchin kata.*"

The Importance of Sanchin　三戦の重要性

空手の動作は独特なもので普段の日常生活や日常的に使う動きではないため型に
よって正しい姿勢、体の極め、呼吸、等、空手に必要な筋肉が要求されます。
特に那覇手系である三戦の型は空手の基本中の基本であり、昔からこの型が出来
れば空手が出来るといわれています。また昔から空手は三戦に始まり三戦に終わ
るという言い伝えが有り、しかも空手をやる者は一日三回この型を鍛錬しらけれ
ばならないとされている。

Karate is made up of movements that we do not ordinarily do in daily life. It is therefore necessary to study the correct posture, the use of fixed poses, breathing techniques and more, in order to develop physique necessary for perform karate.

The very basic *kata* in Okinawa-style karate is *sanchin,* and it has been understood historically that you master karate only if you master this *kata.*

There is also a saying that karate begins with *sanchin* and ends with *sanchin,* and karate fighters should practice *sanchin* every day, three times.

Why is Sanchin Important? なぜ重要か？

空手の姿勢をつくる。戦いにおいては最も安定した姿勢が求められます。
どこから攻撃されても崩れず、また反撃出来る姿勢です、そして最も三戦におい
て重要なのは丹田力があります。そもそも丹田力とは人間の力の中心である処
と武道では言っておりますが、これが使えないとただ筋力だけでは体の大きい
者に負けてしまいます。これは独特の呼吸と正しい姿勢が合体して大きな力とな
るわけです。したがってこれが使えるようになるといくら年をとっても十分に戦
えるわけです。空手にあった体ずくりとは、ただ筋力だけでなくバネのような体
を作らなければ空手はつかえません。ウエイトリフティングによる筋肉ずくり
はかえって逆効果になってしまいます。昔の侍がウエイトリフティングをしたと
云う記録は皆無であります。かえってそのような筋肉は体の動きを遅くしてしま
います。

Karate posture is created by the *sanchin kata*. It is important to have a stable posture when fighting. A practitioner has to be able to stand firm when attacked, and be ready to attack back. The most important aspect in the *sanchin* posture is the power of *Tanden*, which is the central strength in a practitioner. A practitioner will lose to a bigger fighter if only muscle strength is used, and not the *Tanden* power.

Power is created in a combination of correct respiratory breathing and correct posture, which creates tension. It is therefore possible to continue fighting and practicing strong karate as you get older, when this *kata* is used. A physique strengthened from karate is not created only from muscle strength, but from a flexible muscle tone. It is not possible to perform strong karate without this characteristic. A body strengthened with bodybuilding will have an adverse effect. There are no historical documents describing weightlifting among samurai soldiers. Bodies with hard muscles will slow the karate movements of the body.

Mental Preparations When Practicing Sanchin 三戦を稽古するための心構え

そもそも日本の武道において（心、技、体、）の一致をめざす事が最も重要とされている。常に心は平常心を心がけ、いかなる時でも平常と同じ心で行動しなければならない。戦いに挑む時、心が乱れていては、平常の実力は発揮できなません、この平常心を養う方法が三戦呼吸法である。そして次は技であるが、全て技をかける時、極めがなければ中途半端な技になってしまう。正しい技は正しい姿勢によって作られる。正しい姿勢は背筋を伸ばし顎を引き肩をおとし脇をしめいかなる方向からでも倒されない姿勢を作る事である。最後に体、空手における体とはただ単に力や筋肉があるだけでは不十分であり、骨格の構造を利用し、理にかなった動きとバネに似た筋力が求められる。この体をつくるには三戦の型を繰り返し鍛える他は無い。　　　　　　　　　　　　　　　　伊東　博夫

Important elements of martial arts (*Budo*) are the combination of mind, body, and spirit. The mind should be in a stable normal state, and actions should always be taken in a stable mental state. It is not possible for a peak performance if the mind is unstable when preparing for a fight. The respiratory technique of *sanchin* is how you learn to stay stable. The attempt to fight will be half hearted if the technical aspect of *sanchin* has not been mastered. The beginning of a correct technique is correct posture, which is to straighten the spine, pull in the chin, and tilt pelvis up. This posture will enable you to receive blows from any angle. In order to build a body for karate fighting, you do not only build muscle strength, but make use of the bone structure in order to use logical movements and flexibility from muscles. It is therefore vital to repeat training of *sanchin* in order to build a body for karate.

— *by Hiroo Ito*

空手における心構え

人にうたれず人うたず事なきことをもととするなり。
　　　　　　　　　　　　　　　　宮城長順[1]

The spirit of karate
Not to attack, and not being attacked
Act as if there is no fight
— *Chojun Miyagi*

Thoughts on Hiroo Ito's Words
by Kris Wilder

The richness of knowledge presented in the *sanchin kata* is a treasure that has been lost or limited to a very few for a long time. To discover this treasure, we must challenge ourselves to participate in the *kata* as it was originally intended. As we do so, we will certainly find that *sanchin kata* is a far cry from the modern form of karate as practiced by most today.

The tradition was that a person learned one, maybe two forms, or *kata*, and then *sanchin kata* or at least that is the legend. Each *kata* was examined from three perspectives—mind, body, and spirit. Using this method of examination with *sanchin kata*, let us first consider the mind. The very act of practicing *sanchin kata* changes the way the one looks at karate and fighting. Once the practitioner gains the realization of what fighting truly is—the power and damage that can occur—the mind of the practitioner changes. Now, let us consider the body, which experiences change as well. This physical aspect of *sanchin kata* is the most sought after aspect of training in this *kata*. Oddly, it is the easiest of the three to achieve. The *sanchin kata* posture is not like that of the typical Western body, with its broad shoulders and tightly strung muscles. It is, in fact, unattractive by Western standards—the crunched down and rolled shoulders of *sanchin kata* at first glance imply an aged or infirm body. However once the strength of *sanchin kata* is trained and understood, the body will choose this physical position over the classic Western position of shoulders held high, chest puffed out and leaning up on the balls of the feet. Finally, the spirit is changed when the mind comprehends what it is truly doing with respect to fighting, the body begins to adjust to its *sanchin kata* structure posture, and the resulting increased power and speed begin to show themselves. This change can best be described as the kind of spirit an adult would demonstrate to a child who was attempting to fight or cause injury to the adult. The adult understands the situation in a different way and as a result behaves differently—their intent, their spirit, is not the same as the child's.

To the classic practitioner of *sanchin kata*, none of these perspectives—mind, body, or spirit—excludes the others. Some difficulty in understanding *sanchin kata* comes from the source of the *kata*. Although there is no one fountainhead, the language barrier is the largest of these founts of misunderstanding. Chinese, translated to *hogen*, to Japanese, then to English, with regional dialects at each juncture and translations of translations makes for a difficult transfer of accurate information and knowledge.

The importance of what appears to be the simplest of *kata* should not be overlooked because *sanchin kata* forms the hub from which all other *kata* radiate. It is not important as to whether a *kata* was created before or after *sanchin* because *sanchin kata* holds within in it certain undeniable truths. A useful analogy for the relationship of *sanchin kata* to the other *kata* of a given system is that of a bicycle wheel—with *sanchin kata* as the hub and the other *kata* as spokes. The hub must be precisely at the center of the wheel or the wheel functions poorly. It must be made of very good metal to withstand countless rotations over a lifetime of use. A poorly cast or inferior quality metal will fail under stress and usage resulting in the feeble support of the outer rim of the wheel and the eventual collapse of the entire structure. To continue that analogy, when a person looks at a bicycle wheel, the main things they notice are the tire and the spokes. The untrained person will just look at the tire, the most basic and elementary aspect of the bike rather than the structure behind it, the spokes and hub that makes the tire solid." However, to the skilled craftsman who makes a living tuning bicycle wheels, the spokes and the hub are the greatest concern. A spoke that is too taut or too loose will, over time, create damage to the rim on which the tire rests and cause undue stress on the hub. It is also clear that without the hub, the bicycle wheel would turn into a jumbled mess of spokes, collapsed wheel rim, and rubber tire.

Sanchin kata is given a place of honor and respect within the many karate systems that use it, yet it is often not explained, taught, or examined with the intensity and depth required to gain better understanding. For those who practice *sanchin kata*, the impact of the techniques inside this book will be immediate and positive. For those who do not practice *sanchin kata*, there is still much to be gained in understanding body mechanics and application of techniques found within this most universal and comprehensive form. *The Way of Sanchin Kata* illustrates long-overlooked techniques and principles that when applied will radiate throughout your karate, making it more powerful and effective than you will have thought possible.

Preface

No one ever attains very eminent success by simply doing what is required of him; it is the amount and excellence of what is over and above the required that determines the greatness of ultimate distinction.

—Charles Francis Adams [2]

The Way of Sanchin Kata: The Application of Power, will set you on a new course of *sanchin kata* practice. This path of training is overarching and will ultimately buttress your techniques at their very core, making your *kata* and fighting more robust and effective regardless of your level of experience, or *kata* practiced.

Sanchin kata is not like other *kata* in that it stands alone, different and unique. It simply is not cut from the same cloth of other *kata*. In the past, karate masters learned *sanchin kata* and maybe one or two other forms. This way of instruction formed the core of the empty-hand martial arts from the Ryukyu archipelago. The reasoning was clear and uncomplicated: understand the context of empty-hand fighting through *sanchin kata* and learn the content of a fight with other forms.

Today's understanding of the human body exceeds the knowledge of the past immeasurably. Whether modern Western medicine with its magnetic resonance scans, or the revisions and additions made in the East to Traditional Chinese Medicine, the human mind continues to change and adapt increased physiological understanding to today's world.

The basics and practices contained in this manuscript in the past have been buried in "family hands." The techniques, methods, strategies, and tactics were held closely and only passed down from father to son or trusted student. The reasoning behind this veil of secrecy was that once properly trained and with practice, a person could maim another in an instant changing their lives forever. In today's world, a torn medial collateral ligament means surgery and rehabilitation. In six weeks, the knee is functional if not normal again. For most of human history, the same injury may have meant death, or most certainly a diminished life. This helps to explain the primary reason for the veil of secrecy and trust needed to impart this kind of knowledge from teacher to student in the past.

The famous magician Penn Jillette has said to the effect that magicians do not tell how a magic trick is done, which frustrates many people. However, if you really want to know, you can go down to your local magic shop and for twenty dollars, they will sell you the trick and even show you how to do it. Nevertheless, people do not do that because it requires effort, and practice.

Although very different in their goals and methods, magic and *sanchin kata* share a commonality of effort—they both take effort, discipline, and a discerning mind to become good.

This book brings the worlds of modern information and ancient wisdom together. By focusing on the methods of the past masters and proving that knowledge via modern methods, the nature of *sanchin kata* can more readily understood.

This book is not about changing the fundamentals of *sanchin kata*, it is about using the modern mind to gain understanding of the wisdom from the past and to view the wisdom with a modern mind. No matter what the practitioner's goals— enhanced mechanical understanding, advanced mental practice, or a deep spiritual discipline—this book explains it directly and points the way explicitly.

The Way of Sanchin Kata: The Application of Power, will ultimately put *sanchin kata* in terms for the reader that not only dispels mistaken methods but also provides an accurate methodology.

Introduction

There is a principle which is a bar against all information, which is proof against all argument, which cannot fail to keep, and in everlasting ignorance. That principle is condemnation before investigation.

—Edmund Spenser [3]

The Separation of Body, Mind, and Spirit

This book will illustrate the complex and sometimes controversial aspects of *sanchin kata*, a traditional karate form with a rich and varied history. To do that, it is necessary to discuss the cultural precepts that lie in its core. Among these is a holistic view of mind, body, and spirit, a view that is not typically held in the Western world. It was not until recent times that people made such a distinction between the three elements. This distinction or separation of body, mind, and spirit did not happen overnight. In the Western world, it can be traced to several sources, but the primary source in Western thought is René Descartes.[4]

Descartes, the French philosopher, changed the relationship between philosophy and theology when he exclaimed, "I think therefore I am." At that point, Descartes brought about the separation of the mind from the body. Allopathic medicine or Western medicine is firmly rooted in this mind-body separation. To its credit, it is arguably the most successful form of medicine ever known for treating trauma. It achieves this success with a combination of many factors such as pharmacology and a sophisticated physiological understanding of the body.

However, Western medicine, as a guideline, separates the injury from the injured. If you look at a modern operating room, you can see that in many instances, the surgeon cannot see the patient's face. In fact, the entire body except for the area of the operation is covered. Clearly part of this has to do with sanitation and focus, but the obvious representation of the separation of the body from injury should be noted. While this is not a condemnation of Western medicine, it demonstrates a key difference from the way medicine is practiced in the East. Having personally experienced great pain from a viral infection and having modern medicine reduce the fever, deadening the pain in a matter of moments, I would certainly vouch for the benefits of Western medicine. Nevertheless, the understanding of the mind/body/spirit connection is critical in discussing and subsequently understanding *sanchin kata* because *sanchin kata* originated in the East, from a community that used and still uses holistic medicine. *Sanchin kata* is not well suited to being broken down in a Western, deductive reasoning method because of the inherent interaction of the body, the mind, and the spirit.

Of course, these are broad statements used to illustrate a thought and not all examples fit into neat boxes. The same is true of Traditional Chinese Medicine. This discipline seeks harmony of the elements, as do other disciplines such as Ayurvedic medicine, practices that have achieved growth in understanding and acceptance in the West over the past years. *Sanchin kata* can bring these worlds, East and West together. *Sanchin kata* offers a compelling illustration of these Eastern precepts, aiding the practitioner in unifying the body, mind, and spirit, helping to connect with the earth and bring a balance to one's existence.

A simple example of this balance would be the feet. Most of the day, our feet are inside of our shoes, save for when we are bathing or sleeping. Being in shoes is not necessarily a bad thing, but it creates a physical separation from a part of your body, which is not healthy in the long run. The feet become weak and function merely as appendages rather than full participants in the locomotion of our bodies. While performing *sanchin kata* in bare feet, tendons and muscles are activated that are simply not exercised while wearing shoes. In addition, a connection to the earth is achieved, especially when done on the bare ground or a wooden floor. Today it is possible to go a day, even a month without touching the earth unless you seek it. Some people live in an apartment, ride an elevator, walk on concrete ride in a car, park in a garage, sit at a desk, and repeat the process at least five days a week. This is not the way the human body is mean to exist. Movement, breath, and action are an important part of the very existence of a person. *Sanchin kata* incorporates movement, breath, and action, but does it in a way that focuses on self-defense as well.

Generally, the musculature of the body is moved during *sanchin kata* in ways that are not common in the modern world. Taking control of a muscle group, actively with your mind, and with deliberation moving that muscle group is not as common as you might think and is not done while watching television, sitting at a desk, or riding in a car.

Because there are many versions of *sanchin kata* in existence, there are also numerous differing opinions about the execution and meaning of its movements. Opinions and interpretations are often influenced by such factors as 'tribal thinking,' where points of view are kept intact out of allegiance to a person or group, or sometimes an unrealistic adherence to preservation of a form that borders on stagnation. Over the years, different versions of *sanchin kata* have arisen, many of which are in use today. Even within the same systems or styles, one will find differences. Some versions of the form include one-hundred-and-eighty-degree turns. Other versions of the *kata* have no turns. The placement of hands, the speed, and rhythm vary from teacher to teacher depending on what version of the form one chooses to practice. Some of the versions are misplaced in their emphasis. Nobody, when given a choice, would choose the second best when it comes to their karate, their church, or clubs to which they belong. However, sometimes choices are exercised—not by free will, but by example or pressure from peers. For example, my father preferred Chevrolets when it came to cars and, influenced by my father's preference, my choice was the same for years. The reason he liked them was at that time he was able to work on his car, a fact that with today's sophisticated models would no longer hold true. Add to this that in our small town the only dealership was a Chevrolet dealership, a ready resource for parts and that my father worked for the dealership—the preference then makes a world of sense. Following my father's lead, if you had asked me as a young man what I preferred I would have stated, "Chevrolet," without hesitation or thought. Moreover, if you asked me why, I would have said because, "They are the best." Today, while I have a car that I do not work on, live in a major metropolitan city rife with every make and model of car, and do not owe any allegiance to my employer, I still find I hold a preference for a Chevrolet. Tribal allegiances can be very difficult to understand let alone break. The bottom line is it is hard sometimes to break the ties of tribalism, history, and perceptions without deep thought and sense of purpose.

Another factor influencing choice is "preservation." Often times the word, preservation is used in the world of karate leading people to feel like karate should be placed in a jar and placed in the root cellar like fall fruit. Webster's Dictionary lists preservation as "To keep safe from injury, harm, or destruction." Another story from my childhood to illustrate a point is that of the fall ritual of preserving fruit and vegetables. During my childhood, every fall my aunt and my mother would do the season's canning, or preserving, working in the kitchen over cucumbers, peaches, pears and other fruits and vegetables as they came ripe in the garden. Preserving was of course done in preparation for the winter to ensure that we had vegetables and fruits for the winter months. However if given the choice between the fresh peach off the tree that fall or the preserves, I think we would all choose the fresh peach.

A practitioner of *sanchin kata* should preserve the form, protect it from injury or harm, but the student must also be balanced with keeping the form vibrant like the fall peach. To continue the analogy, both the *kata* and the peach should be hanging from the tree limb ripe and colorful. They should not be blanched of their color and syrup added to create a false flavor to make up for the natural flavor now removed—preserved, as fruit placed in a jar.

To that end, it is important to make the distinction between striving to gain the skills of one's teacher and trying to be the teacher. An adherence to just doing what has been done before and presented to you, not having critical thought process for and of one's self will ultimately lead to disappointment. It is said that one may choose to have twenty experiences or the same experience twenty times. At a certain point, one must, without exception, find their own way. In the *Goju Ryu* system of which I am most familiar, the originator or person who standardized of what became *Goju Ryu* karate, Chojun Miyagi[5] made changes to *sanchin kata*. Miyagi took the open hands of the form and closed them to fists. Miyagi then took out the turns in the form his instructor Kanryo Higashionna[6] taught to create another version of the *kata*. Miyagi also changed the breathing taught to him making it more direct and less circulatory in nature.[7] Jigoro Kano,[8] the founder of judo took the principles of the *jiu-jitsu* he had learned as a young man, removed the crippling techniques, created rules for competition, and emphasized throws. Gichin Funakoshi[9] changed his native karate from an Okinawa tradition into a Japanese way to better suit the needs of the Japanese mainland culture. Morihei Ueshiba[10] created *aikido* from his experience with *jiu-jitsu* after an epiphany. Today all of them are cited as masters without question. The list of people changing their art to suit their needs more closely and the needs of their students extends well beyond these examples given. The changes made by these three masters are profound. They were not made without going through a very clear process of gathering the data, analyzing the information, and then making the leap to wisdom. The path to wisdom in these instances has three phases: data, information, and wisdom—each of which has their own unique attributes. In describing those attributes, let us start at the smallest and initial phase: data. The nature of data is that we have no perspective about what it is our how it relates to anything else. Imagine the letter "V" with a line through the middle of the letter, "⊻". Now it is not a letter at all, it is a "⊻", it is data. We have no way to determine value or meaning to this symbol. The data has no position in relation to anything. It is not known where or from whom the data came, what made it, or how it relates to anything. Information, the next piece in the progression, is based on context or how the data relates to other data. Once you have determined the relationship among the data, you have information, a pattern. Turn the "⊻" upside down and you have the letter "A". Now we have relation. We can see that it is the first letter of our alphabet and it makes sense to us now. Wisdom comes from observation of pattern in context of experience, and then a judgment can be made. It is as if we were in English class staring at the upside down letter "A" and someone turned the paper right side up for us. The person turning the letter around for us used their wisdom to recognize the letter and gave us means to comprehension.

Real World Example

A real world example of data, information, and wisdom is the story of my father and a marble. My brother and I were riding in my father's truck up on a plateau above a popular fishing lake in our hometown on a summer day. He pointed to a grove of trees on the plateau. We drove over to the trees, the only ones that I could see for any distance. If my father had not pointed them out, I would have thought nothing of them. When we got out of the truck, I could see old grey wood, which had once been a house, collapsed upon itself. It became clear that it was a homestead. I was in awe that someone had lived there. My mind went wild with the idea that someone lived all the way up here with no roads and no stores. In amazement, I asked my father as he began to walk around how he knew this was here. He explained that a grove of trees in a circle when no other trees are around usually means water and trees grow naturally around water, or somebody planted them. If you have a circular planting of trees, you usually have both water and a homestead because people planted trees for shade. He continued to walk around looking at the ground, then noticing something, knelt down, and called us over as he scratched the ground and pulled out a small clay ball about the size of a dime. Holding it between his thumb and forefinger, he pronounced, "No holes in it." He dropped it in his palm and began to roll it around, noting, "It's not a bead, boys, it's a marble." He went on to say, "It was made by a kid, it is a hand-made marble." My brother and I stood there in the weekend summer sun mesmerized by this thought. A marble made by a kid that has probably already lived and died. My father stood up and put it in his pocket. "These folks probably had a kid or more." My father had applied wisdom based on experience to see the trees, their unique structure, what they most likely meant, and upon exploration found a small clay marble in the dirt made by an unknown child who was part of an unknown family. This is the application of wisdom to understand the context of a pattern and enter into that pattern to find the richness that wisdom can provide.

Kano, Miyagi, Ueshiba, Funakoshi all applied wisdom and inspiration to the information at hand and created living, growing arts.

It is important for practitioners to use the knowledge their instructors have passed on, exercising wisdom and one's life experience. Finally, one must preserve, but not entomb a *kata*. Rather, look to what the *kata* is saying and act accordingly.

This book is not the complete and comprehensive work on *sanchin kata*, it cannot be. The layers, versions and the very nature of *sanchin kata* make it impossible to cover in one book because the form is both deep and broad. A person wishing to integrate *sanchin kata* into their training and essentially their life will find the answer in the application of the principles herein. It is always in the doing. It is always in the experience that true understanding takes place.

CHAPTER ONE

The History of Sanchin Kata

History is the version of past events that people have decided to agree upon.

—Napoleon [11]

The true history of *sanchin kata* is lost to time. Many will claim they know the true and correct history of *sanchin kata,* but factors such as where one chooses to begin and end can create one of many versions of the same history. The goal of this book is to achieve a better understanding of *sanchin kata* through the mechanics, history, and applications of the *kata.* However, the viewpoints between the versions of the history of *sanchin kata* are difficult to make clear. It is only possible to touch upon a handful of points on the timeline with reasonable assurance when looking at the history of *sanchin kata.* Finding the root, or the clear origin, of *sanchin kata* is as difficult as it was for the British and French in 1854 to find the headwaters of the Nile River.

When a person chooses to begin in a different place or, say, with particular instructor, and move backward a different length of time, you have a different history. Just as an explorer, seeking the headwaters of the Nile River, had to make choices when the waters forked, changing the path of the exploration, every student of *sanchin kata* serves as a fork in the flow of history.

For example, in the southern states of the United States of America the title, "The War of Northern Aggression" is used to describe the Civil War. Was the westward expansion in the United States truly a "Manifest Destiny" or a land grab combined with genocide? Again, one's perspective determines their outlook or conclusion.

Oral history is by its nature fallible, the following is a version of the history of *sanchin kata*; again, a history, not the only history.

A Buddhist[12] holy man named Bodhidharma[13] is credited with leaving India in 539 A.D. to spread the Buddhist faith to China. He left his monastery in Southern India not knowing that he was going to spread Buddhism in a most unique way. Bodhidharma traveled enormous distances compared to the people of his time who were born, lived, and died in and around their home village or city. He crossed the

Himalayan Mountains and the Yangtze River on his way to the capital of the Henan Province, located in the eastern part of what is China today, halfway between the northern border with Mongolia and the southern border of the South China Sea. Bodhidharma arrived at the Shaolin Temple. It is unclear if the Shaolin temple was his destination or simply a stopover to another place. Nevertheless, it became a profound juncture in martial arts history.

During Bodhidharma's time, people often would come to the temple for many reasons, hunger and shelter to name a few. Many were turned away. After several attempts to enter the temple, Bodhidharma, an Indian foreigner was finally admitted. It is said that at this point he found the Shaolin monks weak from lack of physical activity. It seems that the monks spent so much time in meditation that their bodies had been neglected. Bodhidharma introduced his methods of exercise that began to change the physiology of the monks and strengthen their bodies. These exercises changed over time and became part of the now famous practice of Shaolin *kung fu*.

Now let us jump ahead some eight hundred years where, as Chinese tradition has it, part of the *sanchin kata* history can be traced to a 13th century priest. Zhang San Feng began his martial arts instruction with the Shaolin monks. He learned the external, or hard, methods that involved strengthening the body through repetitions of techniques and the use of other items like bags full of sand or rock serving as rough dumbbells, striking poles, and other means to bring more power to his *kung fu*. At some time in his training, Zhang San Feng left the temple. The reason given is he felt he had learned all he could and needed to explore other means. Whatever the reason, the story has it his next destination was on the Wutang Mountain at a temple called the Purple Summit Temple. The Purple Summit Temple was said to be among the most sacred Taoist Monasteries at the top of the Earth suspended between Heaven and Earth.

At this time, he is said to have seen a snake and crane fighting and was moved by their fluidity and power of their movements. With this inspiration, Zhang San Feng set out to recreate what he had learned in this new environment. Over time, the hard (external) methods of his previous training gave way to softer internal methods of training. His system was soon known as *Wutang Lohan Chuan-fa*,[14] or thirty-two pattern long fist. He taught this system to his students and over time, the forms underwent a drastic metamorphosis into *Tai Chi Chuan-fa*, or Grand Ultimate. Today there are many forms of *Tai Chi Chuan-fa* and the major forms Chen, Yang, and Wu are named after the families who propagated their particular version.

Over time, the martial and health attributes of *Tai Chi Chuan-fa* became more widely known. In the same fashion, Zhang San Feng had changed what he had learned to suit his needs and the forms continued to change as his students changed what they were taught to better suit their needs.

The next leap we make in time is from the 13th century to the 20th century and some six hundred years where according to the history of the *Goju Ryu* lineage, Kanryo Higashionna (1853-1915)[15] brought *sanchin kata* back to Okinawa. That is not to say that *sanchin kata* had not been introduced to Okinawa before. It simply means the version that Higashionna brought back was taught by him to students who propagated the form by teaching it to others. Around 1918, Kanbun Uechi[16] brought another version of *sanchin kata* to Okinawa and began teaching what would later be known as *Uechi Ryu*. As the reader can see, many paths for martial arts, as well as many paths for *sanchin kata* can be identified. Tracing that history involves a great deal of sifting through a rich mix of history, mythology, legend, and cultural prejudices often indistinguishable from one another. That is why nobody knows for sure about the origins of *sanchin kata*.

These many paths of course, are a result of change—both deliberate and accidental—to the practice of *sanchin kata*. Some might argue that in the case of martial arts and its forms, change is bad. On the contrary, the key to the concept of change is context. If change is a result of suiting the needs of the practitioner enacting the change, it may well be credible. However, change can result from mistranslation of a movement, or a misunderstanding of the intent behind a form or an element. While some changes are credible, e.g., are made consciously to suit one's needs, others are accidental. An analogy might be the children's game "telephone." The game is a simple one. While sitting in a circle, one person whispers a phrase into the ear of the person next to them and the message goes around the circle until the last person says what they were told and compares it to the originator's words. With few exceptions, does the phrase ever come out at the end in the same way it originated? This phenomenon is not unique to this game nor is it unique to the martial arts. Even some of our most sacred texts are misquoted. The Bible for example reads in 1st Timothy 6:10 "For the love of money is the root of all evil."[17] That phrase has often been misquoted as "Money is the root of all evil," a distinct difference. Then there are just the accidental changes, the result of simply being human. A wonderful example of this is "Spoonerism,"[18] a term named after W.A. Spooner (1844-1900), an English clergyman noted for the transposition of the letters of two words often resulting in gibberish. An example of a Spoonerism is, "Sleepy time becomes Teepy slime."[19] I am confident that you have had many conversations where you have transposed, left out, or added a word that may have made you all laugh at the result. The point is that no means of information transference that involves the human mind, with all its prejudgments, or assumptions, is exact.

As changes, accidental or deliberate, take place, in some instances the forms become more simplified and in others more complicated. Soon many paths are created. For example, there are versions of *sanchin kata* that face in only one direction during the performance of the *kata* never turning. Some versions of *sanchin kata* turn. Some versions have opened hands and others have closed hands. Some submit that closing the fist closes off the *ki* (or *chi*) and others would say it makes the *kata* stronger turning the *ki* back into the practitioner.

The book, *Five Ancestor Fist Kung-Fu, The Way of Ngo Cho Kun* by Alexander L. Cho offers a straightforward path of *sanchin kata* through the *kung fu* system, "The *kata* taught by Miyagi[20] are the *sanchin kata* and *tensho*. The *sanchin kata* of *Goju Ryu* is notably similar in principles and movements to the *sam chien* of *Ngo Cho Kun*. The movements and principles of the *tensho kata* are also strikingly similar to *Ngo Cho Kun*, and it seems the similarities are by no means coincidental. *Uechi Ryu*, another major Okinawan karate style, also bears striking resemblance to *Ngo Cho Kun*."

Taijiquan (Tai Chi Chuan), The Grand Ultimate Fist, is often considered one of the three sisters of *kung fu*: *Hsing-I, Baguazhang*, and *Tai Chi Chuan*. *Tai Chi* is often taught in the western world as a form of health exercise but it is also a devastating martial art when employed in the hands of a knowledgeable practitioner. The very beginning of one *Tai Chi* segment, "Grasping the Sparrow's Tail," looks very similar to the opening of *sanchin kata*.[21] *Ngo Cho Kun*, the Five Ancestor Fist *kung fu* uses a *kata* called *sam chin* and the similarities between the Okinawan version of *sanchin kata* and the Chinese version of *sam chin* are not coincidental. The fact of the latter is that the Okinawan version of *sanchin kata*, no matter what the school or *ryu*, derives from forms originating from mainland China.

Again, the work of uncovering, deciphering, and contextualizing historical information is a task that must involved educated speculation where contradictions, limited and unreliable source material and other hurdles exist. The goal is to present probable conclusions where possible, and to raise compelling questions where the truth has been lost to time.

Regardless of which system one chooses, what matters is that certain constants are necessary for success, 'success' being defined as:

1. **Gripping the ground.** This is interpreted as using the ground to generate power in holding one's position or striking power.
2. **Skeletal architecture.** The alignment of the bones to provide static strength.
3. **Muscular tone.** Using conditioned muscles to move the body swiftly and in a way beneficial to the technique being done.
4. **Moving the ki (universal energy).** Using intent and bioelectric energy to assist in movement.
5. **Calming the mind to mushin, or "no mind."** Removing internal chatter to allow the mind to function more efficiently.

Chapter Two

Learning by Emulation and Repetition

I hear and I forget. I see and I remember. I do and I understand.

—*Confucius* [22]

The two fundamental parts of learning are emulation and repetition. The way in which these are done makes a big difference in the level of success that a person acquiring a new skill experiences. Writing is an excellent example of this method of emulation and repetition. The teacher writes on the board a letter and the students copy the letter on their own paper. The letter when first shown is basic in its style. In the case of the English language, the letter would no doubt be written in an upper case and block fashion. The letter "A" would be explained with the first stroke as, "Start at the top and move down like this and "/" the second stroke of the pen is the other side, "\" and finally the horizontal line "-" all together comprising an "A". The next letter would then be introduced and so on until the entire alphabet was covered. Lower case letters would follow the process then starting over. Once the letters are learned, words can be introduced and assembled. Sentences are next, small ones at that, and paragraphs, small to large and so on. After a while, as the student matures, the writing becomes more personal and in some instances almost illegible. During this process, nerve pathways are built, some re-enforced, and in some instances, other old nerve endings are allowed by the body to atrophy as new connections supersede and replace the old connections. This rewiring is often described as muscle memory. Muscle memory is also what is needed in combat. The Romans spent an enormous amount of time, upwards of two years, drilling new recruits in the use of the shield, sword, and battlefield maneuvers before they ever saw real battle. This pattern of training, systematic and standardized, created the greatest army known to man at the time and sustained the Pax Romana for two centuries. The idea of muscle memory and discipline are not new to man and in fact are as old at civilized man himself, only the name is recent.

Sanchin kata provides the repetition in a mechanical form to achieve the muscle memory needed to perform in a stress situation. The brilliance of *sanchin kata* from the mechanical standpoint is that it slows down the movements of the body. This slowing down of the movements permits the practitioner to learn in a manner that is known today as the demonstration phase of the education process. The student can actually see what happens in the smallest detail. The student sees the demonstration, then begins to emulate the motion slowly improving on the action, and almost without perception moves to the next phase of learning, integration. Through demonstration, emulation, and integration, the motion and the student become one.

Chapter Three

The Mechanics of Being in the Moment

That moves and that moves not,
That is far and the same is near.
That is within and all this and
That is also outside all this.

—Isha Upanishad [23]

In today's films, a popular technique is to slow a motion down to give emphasis to the action in the film. The point of slowing the scene down is that it allows us to take in the nuances of the event. In the scientific world, super high-speed film is used in experiments ranging from seeing how a hummingbird flies and to the impact of an automobile into a test structure during impact safety studies. The creators of *sanchin kata* knew of this learning process far before the invention of high-speed film. *Sanchin kata* breaks down the movements into the incremental principles that need to be understood to gain the skills necessary to become proficient at the art of the empty hand.

Sanchin is translated as "three battles" or difficulties. The accepted three are mind, body, and spirit. The difficulty is bringing these three together at one time and in one place. A question that one might want to ask is why should I want to bring these three together? The answer is that if a person is functioning at the physical level then they are nothing more than an animal. That is to say, they have no ability to control what it is their instincts tell them to do.

The Brain and its Elements

The hemispheres of the cerebral cortex are divided in half from front to back into the right hemisphere and the left hemisphere. Each hemisphere specializes in some tasks and behaviors. The hemispheres communicate with each other via the corpus callosum, a thick band of 200-250 million nerve fibers. The corpus callosum serves as the telephone company that services these two sections of the brain allowing communication.

The right side of the brain controls muscles on the left side of the body and the left side of the brain controls muscles on the right side of the body. In general, sensory information from the left side of the body crosses over to the right side of the brain and information from the right side of the body crosses over to the left side of the brain. Therefore, brain damage to one side of the brain will affect the opposite side of the body.

In 95% of right-handers, the left side of the brain is dominant for language. Even in 60-70% of left-handers, the left side of brain is used for language. In the 1860s and 1870s, two neurologists Paul Broca and Karl Wernicke observed that when people had damage to a particular area on the left side of the brain, they had speech and language problems. They noticed that people with damage to these specific areas on the right side usually did not have any language problems. The two language areas of the brain that are important for language now bear their names: Broca's area and Wernicke's area.

Arming the Body

It is important to understand the communication between the two hemispheres of the brain during a threatening event. When a threat is perceived, the amygdala goes to work. The amygdala is the part of your brain located approximately at the underside of the temporal lobe. The amygdala's job is to sound a siren call to action. This means the central nervous system is activated to the threat with an all systems alert. The hypothalamus, which regulates the vitals of the body, triggers the pituitary gland. The pituitary gland, located around the bottom of the brain, produces thyrotropin to stimulate the thyroid gland and adrenocorticotropin (ACTH), a chemical that fires up the adrenal cortex. In other words, the adrenal system shoots adrenaline throughout the body. Non-essential body functions are shut down or reduced. Think of it this way: The body is saying if we do not get through this, nothing else may matter so everything goes to arming the body, and all long-term projects are shut down.

When the adrenaline hits the body, the pupils dilate. They open up to let as much light in to facilitate threat recognition. The eyes, the only exposed part of the brain, relay information to the thalamus. The thalamus acts as the mixing and incorporation superhighway of sensory information blending the sights, sounds, and other sensory intake into terms the brain can understand. The thyroid gland pours thyroglobulin, an iodine-containing protein that increases metabolic rate, into the body and the resting metabolic rate rises. The result is more energy is now available to the body to use as it sees fit.

In the lungs, the bronchioles dilate. The walls of the air pipes in the lungs in essence become larger to allow more air to pass into the lungs. Hair stands on end to give the body a little larger area of sensory reception. The liver breaks down glycogen which is the main form in which carbohydrate is stored in liver tissue. This breakdown of glycogen provides instant energy and helps to keep up with the higher metabolic rate the thyroid has initiated. The spleen, which is an organ located in the left of the abdomen near the stomach concerned with final destruction of red blood cells, and filtration and storage of blood, contracts while pumping out white blood cells to fight infection and platelets that assist in blood clotting. The skin vessels constrict causing sweat and cooling the body as it works above its normal operating limits. Meanwhile the adrenaline has hit the heart and blood pressure rises there as well. The body system is ready to perform, almost.

When the body goes on high alert, all bodily activities that do not have direct association with the fight or flight situation are reduced. The bladder that holds the urine and the colon that holds the feces prepare to void. The body does not need any extra weight and needs to reduce any infectious waste that could present a problem to the body if injured. The stomach and the gastrointestinal tract constrict redirecting blood to the muscles.

Now the body is, to use a military phrase, locked and loaded.[24]

The Hemispheres of the Brain

The right and the left hemispheres of the brain appear to be mirror images of one another, but they have different structures and different roles.

The left hemisphere does an excellent job of seeing words in order and making sense of letters. The left hemisphere deals with logic and the analytical thought processes such as retrieving the number inside the cell of a spreadsheet, but has trouble understanding how that number relates to the spreadsheet in its entirety. The right hemisphere specializes in the recognition and understanding of space, shapes, and forms. The right hemisphere is the creative side of the brain. It can assemble the puzzle and give a number on a spreadsheet meaning.

The point is clear that smooth communication between the two hemispheres of the brain together provides the best viewpoint of the world. When information is absent or communication between the two hemispheres is impeded, the context of the information is destroyed and incorrect decisions can result.

A former military officer and martial artist explained to me one time what he called the "pucker factor." Oddly enough, the pucker factor that takes place is the constriction of the corpus callosum. Because the chemicals that are released into the body during a stress situation, the corpus callosum shrinks in size, contracting making communication between the two hemispheres less easy. The reason for this constriction is as stated before; the lower brain is in charge of fight or flight. The lower brain wants little interference with the process of survival because instinct and action are the markers of the moment, and thinking is for later.

Corpus Callosum

Training of course is the best means of insuring the negative aspects of the pucker factor—the restriction of creativity and logic to interact—has a smaller effect on the body. One of the ways to ensure minimum negative affect of the pucker factor is stimulating the corpus callosum. The corpus callosum, the brain's telephone company, needs to be as communicative as possible. This can be done by using the body to activate the brain.

A good example of where the corpus callosum comes into play can be found in *sambo,* which is a Russian form of combat designed for and by the Russian military to use in close-quarters combat. One day when I was having a conversation with a former world *sambo* competitor and United States Marine Corps combat instructor, I commented that from what I had seen on television (since I had never seen Russians compete in *sambo* live) that they were tough customers. They also seemed to have a genetic predisposition not to feel pain at the same level that others seemed to have. He quickly and calmly looked at me and said, "No, it is just the way they train." After some conversation, it became clear that it was about the way they trained their body, but also the way they trained their minds.

Controlling the brain is important whether you are involved in *sanchin kata,* the military, or any other form of martial arts. There are many forms of controlling and training the brain. One of the most fundamental means of doing this training is understanding the split between the two hemispheres.

Why is this split in the brain important to a practitioner of *sanchin kata?* It has to do with marching, walking, and the way the body operates the brain during these two activities. One activity allows for unification of the brain, walking. The other action, marching, tends to separate communication in the brain and reduces thinking.

Marching is used in today's military as a training tool more than as a practical means of moving an army from one place to another. However, during the majority of military battles prior to the industrial revolution, marching was the chief means of moving an army because efficiency was essential. Marching is different than walking in that it is a same-side body action, left arm, left foot, and then the right arm and right foot swing forward on the other side of the body. When the left side of the body, arm, and foot swing forward, they activate the right side of the brain and the right side activates the left side as discussed earlier. The corpus callosum, the brain's telephone company, is little used. The end result is there is reduced contact between the two hemispheres of the brain. Again, active thinking takes both sides of the brain communicating about the issue before it. Think of thinking as cooking a good stew; it involves meat, potatoes, other vegetables, and the right seasonings. To continue the analogy, marching restricts the making of stew. Marching keeps a group of men in a fixed order while covering distance and also, premeditated or not, keeps them from thinking too much. Walking on the other hand is counterbalancing when it comes to the physical body. Walking is left arm, right foot and right arm left foot. These motions stimulate the opposite side of the brain that is communicated via the corpus callosum.

In applied kinesiology, the Hetero-lateral Neurological Cross Crawl or just Cross Crawl[25] is used to facilitate the communication between the two sides of the brain. The method is as follows: standing naturally facing forward, the subject lifts the right arm so the bicep is parallel to the floor the hand of the same arm is point skyward giving the right arm a ninety-degree bend at the elbow. The opposite leg, the left leg, lifts to mimic the same ninety-degree bends as the arm. The thigh is level with the floor and the calf hangs vertical to the floor. Then the process is switched in a smooth manner as if walking in place. This is repeated some fifteen times. The Cross Crawl fortifies the corpus callosum and tones the connections between the hemispheres of the brain. An analogy would be the difference between an old road and a beautiful new four-lane highway. The new highway allows more traffic at a faster rate because of a better surface and efficient use of passing lanes and High Occupancy Vehicle Lanes (HOV) that the old two lanes simple do not have.

Moving in *sanchin kata*, because it is a walk and not a march, helps create better communication between the two sides of the brain. Often it is said by practitioners

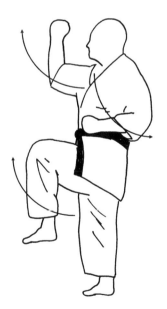
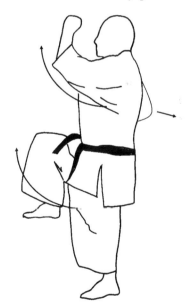

CROSS CRAWL POSITION ONE - RIGHT ARM AND LEFT LEG   CROSS CRAWL POSITION TWO - LEFT ARM AND RIGHT LEG

and instructors of *sanchin kata* that the *kata* is a form of moving meditation. That in doing *sanchin kata* a means is built to bring the three battles, of mind, body, and spirit together and unifying the mind is the ground, the base, the very beginning of the process of unification.

British golfer Tony Jacklin describes the "cocoon of concentration" he sometimes finds himself in: "When I'm in this state, this cocoon of concentration, I'm living fully in the present, not moving out of it. I am aware of every half inch of my swing …I'm absolutely engaged, involved in what I am doing at that particular moment. That's the important thing. That's the difficult state to arrive at. It comes and it goes, and pure fact that you go out on the first tee of the tournament and say, 'must concentrate today,' is no good. It will not work. It has to already be there."[26]

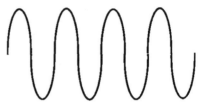

BETA— Actively Awake 14 to 21 pulses per second

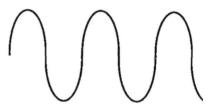

ALPHA— Relaxed Awake 7 to 14 pulses per second

Brain Cycles

As all of the above-mentioned aspects come together, the practitioner enters into the alpha brain wave state. There are four levels of brain activity: beta, alpha, theta, and delta. Brain waves are recorded scientifically by measuring the fluctuating electrical impulses in the brain. Beta waves range from 14 to 30 cycles per second. Such pulses are indicative of a person who is fully awake, alert, excited, or tense. Alpha waves run from 8 to 13 cycles per second. They are characterized by deep relaxation, passive awareness, or a composed state of mind. Theta waves range from 4 to 7 cycles per second. They are indicative of a person who is drowsy, unconscious, or in a state of deep tranquility. Delta waves run from

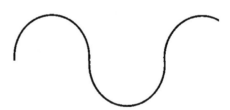

THETA — beginning of sleep 4 to 7 pulses per second

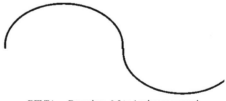

DELTA — Deep sleep 0.5 to 4 pulses per second

THE FOUR BRAIN FREQUENCIES.

0.5 to 3.5 cycles per second. They are characterized by sleep, unawareness, or deep unconsciousness.

The first two levels, beta and alpha, are the ones we are concerned with in martial arts. The brain discharges the beta wave when we are awake and intentionally focused. We are alert, ready for action, even irritated or afraid. This is because we are looking at the active mind. Beta is not as useful as alpha is to the martial artist. In a nutshell, beta is about thinking and thinking quite frequently gets you hit.

The alpha state is indicative of physical and mental relaxation, the relaxed, but alert mind. It is usually achieved during meditation. In the alpha state, we are aware of what is happening around us yet ultra-focused in our concentration. The professional athlete would call it being "in the zone," or being "in the flow." We have all heard of athletes who while facing great impediments to their games, such as the flu, an injury, or another tragedy, have excelled beyond what was expected. A large part of their success and performance directly results from an ability to shift into the alpha state of consciousness during competition.

One of the benefits to training in martial arts is the ability to switch between beta (waking brain waves) and alpha ("the zone") brain waves. Multiple studies have shown that world-class athletes, no matter what the sport, have the ability to move their brain waves almost instantly from beta to alpha. This is also frequently demonstrated by martial artists. Board-breaking techniques are a good example. Concentration begins as the hand moves into chamber. By the time a practitioner's fist strikes a board or the brick, his or her mind is fully in an alpha state. The target shatters effortlessly.

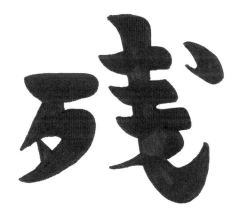

Zanshin

Zanshin means continuing mind. It is a state of enhanced awareness that should exist just before, during, and after combat. A practitioner in this state should be hyper-aware of his or her surroundings and prepared for anything.[27]

Unconsciousness is illustrated in a famous explanation of just how important

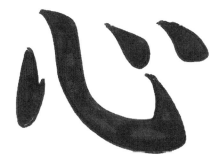

KANJI FOR *ZANSHIN,* CONTINUING MIND.

is this mental state. In his efforts to study Zen archery, German philosopher[28] Eugen Herrigel's Zen master who taught him insisted, "the shot will only go smoothly when it takes the archer himself by surprise…you mustn't open your hand on purpose."[29]

This moving meditation, this continuing mind of *zanshin*, is part and parcel of *sanchin kata*.

Chapter Four

Measurement, Personal and Unique

Everything is arranged according to a number and mathematical shape.

—*Pythagoras* [30]

A friend of mine whom I have known for some twenty-five years is a tracker, that is to say he goes out into the woods and spends time simply observing the wilderness and tracking animals. Having grown up around mountains, creeks, and rivers, it was not a large jump for him to get training in the ways of tracking by Tom Brown, Jr.,[31] the author of many books on the subject.

Looking to experience this myself, I spent three days in and around the woods in eastern Washington with him. After tracking deer and bear, finding dead animals, and learning their stories, we found ourselves on the last day, a Sunday morning, on the edge of a man-made dike. The sandy road that ran alongside of the dike allowed the state access along the river. It had also turned into a wonderful entrance to nature for the locals. We crouched in the early morning sunlight as it broke through the tall pine trees and the lesson began. He pointed to some tracks in the sand. The size and width of the footprint told him it was a woman, the length of the stride and the way the sand kicked up inside the print told him she was exceeding her natural stride. He pointed to the dog paw prints next to her footprints. It was unlikely they were unrelated prints, he explained. Domestic dogs and people take a straight path because they have a destination. In contrast, coyotes and stray dogs, because they are always searching for the next meal, rarely move in a straight line. He again looked at the woman's footprint and stride. He estimated her height, and, pressing his hand into the sand, pronounced her estimated weight. He then repeated the process with the dog tracks. He stopped and said, "Follow me," and we quickly got off the road to stand in a grove of trees. He stood ramrod straight and out of the corner of his mouth he said, "Be a tree." I copied him. Seconds later, to my amazement, a woman matching the description given, walked by us with her dog.

My friend knew that the length of a person's foot corresponds to the length of shin plus a proportion more. As an example, my foot is ten inches long, my shin is fourteen inches long, and my thigh is seventeen inches long. The measurement of the foot, shin, and thigh show they become increasingly larger by about three or four inches or roughly twenty-five percent. This example of the measurements is not a strict adherence to the Fibonacci Ratio[32] because few people have perfect proportions, but is close to the ratio. This demonstrates how my friend, the tracker, upon knowing a person's foot size was in turn able to determine the unseen person's shin measurement. He then related that measurement proportionally to the thigh and other parts of the body allowing him to determine the woman's approximate size and weight. Without my knowing it, I had been introduced to an application of the Fibonacci Ratio via Native American tracking methods.

As a culture inherently in tune with nature, Native Americans are familiar, though not in name, with the Fibonacci Ratio and use it as a tool to make sense of, and to live successfully within, their environment. The creators of *sanchin kata* also applied this ratio to create a training form that was in tune with nature. In both instances, an understanding of this ratio as an underlying principle of nature and applying it to life is critical; failure to do so is a formula for failure.

Fibonacci Ratio

The Fibonacci Ratio was discovered by Leonardo Pisano Fibonacci (1170–1250)[33] Living in Pisa, Italy, he researched and discovered that nature had a structural formula. The formula was named after him and is called the Fibonacci Ratio today. This ratio is found in every natural structure on the planet—plant, animal, and your body as well. It regularly appears in the growth patterns of many living things, such as the spiral formed by a seashell or the curve of a fern. It is, in fact, the only growth pattern that, if continued, is not doomed to failure. Thus, it is a principle of structural integrity. The basics of the ratio can be understood by starting with the number 1. You then add the number 1 by itself, 1+1=2. Then take the result, in this case the 2, and add the preceding number to it so 1+2=3 and begin to repeat the addition so that your number line looks like this, 1, 1, 2, 3, 5, 8, 13, 21, etc.

Another way to understand the Fibonacci Ratio is with shapes. Start with two squares the same size and place them next to each other. These squares represent the number 1. As we did earlier, we started with two 1's and we need to do so again. On top of these, we then draw a square of size 2 where the 2 is equal to 1+1. Now draw a third square on top of the two smaller ones. The third square is equal to the next number in sequence, or 2, 1+1=2. To make the fourth square take the length of the 2 and a 1 square and copy it three times making another square. This fourth square is equal to the 3 number in the number line, 1, 1, 2, 3. Repeating this process creates a visual representation of the Fibonacci Ratio.

The Fibonacci Ratio can be found in your body as well and can be easily found in your hand. Lift up your hand and make a fist. Then lift your index finger up into

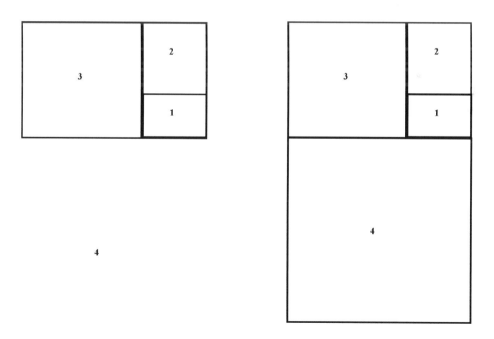

FIBONACCI SQUARE #1

FIBONACCI SQUARE #2

FIBONACCI SQUARE #3

FIBONACCI SQUARE #4

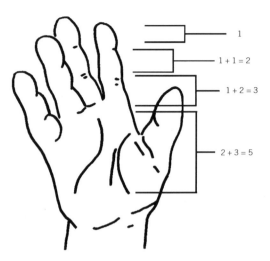

THE FIBONACCI RATIO IN THE HUMAN HAND.

the shape of a hook and look at the tip of your finger to the first knuckle. Consider this tip of your finger to be equal to the primary unit of the Fibonacci formula, the 1. The second joint, slightly longer, is equal to 1+1=2 part of the formula, and the next joint is 1+2=3. The metacarpal bone (any bone on the back of the hand between the wrist and the fingers) is equal to 2+3=5.

This ratio is intimately connected with the Golden Mean, a concept derived by the ancient Greeks and used by them as well as the ancient Egyptians in the design of buildings and monuments such as the Parthenon and the Great Pyramids. While employing the concept of the Golden Mean, the ancients discovered they could create a feeling of natural order as well as structural integrity in their works. Human creations of the Golden Mean are simple to see and prevalent. To see where the ratio shows up in everyday life, all you need to do is open your wallet or purse and look at any credit card and you will see the Golden Mean. Even the design of playing cards is based on the Golden Mean.

Again, because this ratio is among the basic mathematical formulas upon which nature builds, it is important that we acknowledge this and work in harmony with nature, and not against it. Think of it this way; close your eyes and imagine you have everything you need to build a ten-foot-tall pyramid—the stone, the mortar, and a crane. In your mind, take a few seconds and build the pyramid. Now look at it. The point is at the top, correct? Clearly, you cannot build an upside-down pyramid and have it stand. It simply is not stable and tips over to seek a balance point. If you did build a pyramid upside down, you would need supports to hold it in the upside-down position. Those supports, of course, would not be needed if you build the pyramid correctly to begin with. It follows then, that in *sanchin kata*, one should adhere to the ratio. Not to do so is the equivalent of building an upside-down pyramid.

In the martial arts, we do not use feet or meters, we measure using our own body. We use finger widths, fists, and feet (the kind you stand on, not the twelve-inch kind). This allows a person to measure the widths, depths, and heights necessary for the martial arts against their own body. This form of measurement is the same way

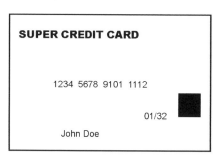

THE FIBONACCI RATIO IN A CREDIT CARD.

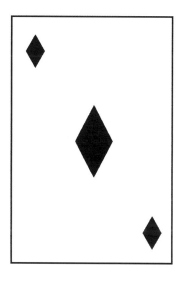

THE FIBONACCI RATIO IN A PLAYING CARD
(ACE OF DIAMONDS).

my tracker friend was able to determine these elements of height, weight, and depth of a person he had not yet seen. Using a personal form of measurement allows the practitioner to tailor the movements of martial arts to suit their physical needs. In Chinese, or Traditional Chinese Medicine, an example of such a form of measurement is a *kua*, the size of your closed fist. The term *kua* is used in the title of *Pa Kua Chang*, or Eight Hand Changes. A *tsun* (pronounced "soon") is the width of your index and middle fingers placed together. Because these measurements are based on a specific body part and not a standard external form of measurement, such as an inch, this is precisely the method that allowed my tracker friend to look at a footprint of a woman he had never seen and determine what her entire body might look like.

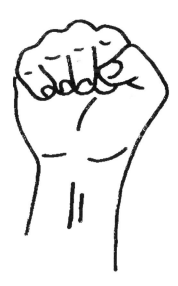

KUA, CANTONESE FOR FIST.

We use this Chinese form of measurement when doing *sanchin kata* and, for that matter, any *kata*. *Sanchin kata* teaches the fundamentals of karate that can then be extended over the entire syllabus of karate. This extension of this principal gives the practitioner the structural integrity of the basics throughout their martial arts techniques.

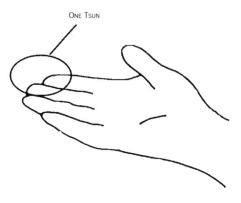

ONE TSUN

TSUN, CANTONESE FOR WIDTH OF TWO FINGERS.

CHAPTER FIVE

The Roots of a Strong Tree, the Feet

Sticks in a bundle are unbreakable.

—*Kenyan Proverb*[34]

A tree grows from the ground up and a practitioner should grow his or her *sanchin kata* in the same way. To continue the analogy, a tree that has strong roots, 'strong' in this case meaning 'deep', will not give way when a storm comes along. Shallow roots or diseased roots guarantee the tree will be blown over in a storm. The same is true in the martial arts. Therefore, it is essential to have a powerful, 'rooted' stance, one that will serve you well today and in later years as well.

The feet should have as much surface area on the ground as possible without rolling the foot to place the arch on the ground, hence collapsing the arch. The foot

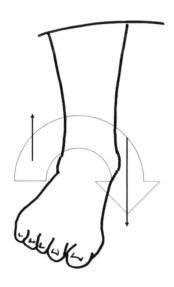

FOOT ROLLED INWARD TOWARD
CENTERLINE OF BODY.

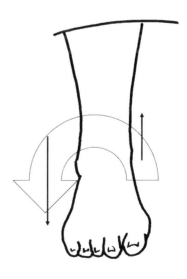

FOOT ROLLED OUTWARD AWAY
FROM CENTERLINE OF BODY.

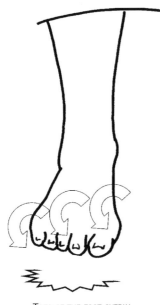

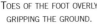

TOES OF THE FOOT OVERLY
GRIPPING THE GROUND.

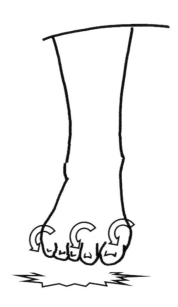

TOES OF THE FOOT GRIPPING THE GROUND.

must remain natural and flattened. Flattening the arch rotates the foot inside and lifts the outside of the foot, reducing the power of the contact to the ground. The foot must be placed on the ground as if it is made of wet clay. It should feel heavy and as if it is gripping the ground, though the toes should not actually be in a gripping position such as if trying to pick up a piece of paper from the floor. To do this uses too much physical power and creates rigidity, and rigidity is easily displaced. Instead, the toes should come into firm contact with the ground and not overly grip.

When you want to move your foot, you simply do it. Moreover, when you need to be rooted to the ground, you are. As simple as that sounds, people can stay rooted during their entire movement. The result is not good—a step that looks as if the practitioner is pulling their foot out of deep mud and slogging it forward to place it in more mud. The goal again is straightforward: when you need to be rooted you are, and when you need to move, move.

The line of the pressure on the foot needs to be from the heel of the foot through the center of the foot. Severely rotating the foot or twisting the foot to gain traction is potentially damaging to the knee farther up the leg. It supinates the foot, placing pressure on the inside of the foot, and taking the weight off the centerline.

Where the circumstances of, or the choices made in, one's life results in the reduction of key body functionality, the body will make compensations. Often, these compensations do not become known until later in life. A man I know who has worked in the music business has significant hearing loss. Years of rock-and-roll concerts and loud music have taken their toll. He always says in a half joking half serious way, "Kids, take care of your hearing." Now his body compensates for his hearing loss by increased reliance on vision. It is helpful to him to look directly at a person when they are speaking to understand what is being said. A body will make numerous similar compensations if it is required.

When performing *sanchin kata*, poor structure in stances will eventually catch up with a person. Just like years of loud rock and roll, the damage may not be apparent at the beginning but it will, without a doubt, manifest itself soon enough. Among the easiest places to see potential damage arising is in the knee joint.

On the positive side, a great example of this kind of innate grounding skill is found in every judo *dojo* in the world. Skilled judo practitioners are able to control their weight and balance easily. It is especially apparent when a practitioner is pitted against one of a significantly lower rank. The junior ranks are simply not able to throw higher ranks even when it appears that the junior has set the technique well against the senior. The senior often counters the junior's technique explosively throwing the junior to the mat.

Clearly, the overmatch of skill is the key here, but the ability of the senior to simply hold their position—in essence

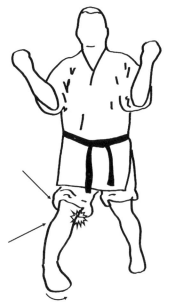

FOOT SEVERELY TWISTED INWARD
VIA KNOCK-KNEED STANCE.

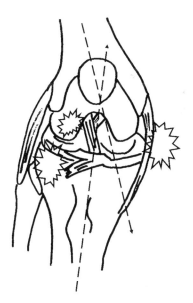

TENDONS OF THE KNEE STRESSED
DURING KNOCK-KNEED STANCE.

gripping the ground and then separate from the gripping action to become swift and explosive instantly—is the point of this example. This is not unique to karate or judo. The ability to control this grounding and explosion is found in many contact sports, in one form or another, and at various levels of intensity in the martial arts.

The footing in *sanchin kata* can be deceptive in its placement. This first illustration shows the foot placement sometimes used by some schools where the rear foot is turned acutely inward, an exaggeration of the twisting inward sensation.

The second illustration shows the foot placement that allows for a refined body structure higher up the body. The centerline of the rear foot is placed forward with

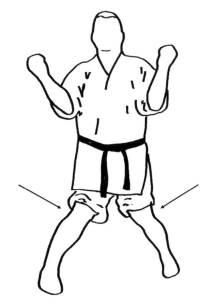

KNEES PINCHED WITH TOES TWISTED INWARD EXAGGERATED-

the centerline running from the heel to the index toe, the largest toe on the foot.

From a front view, it would appear the same right triangle would be used—running down the femur straight down to the ground and then forming the triangle with the shin. This, however, is incorrect because it can compromise the knee. A forensic archaeologist, upon studying a skeleton, can tell a great deal about a person and how he or she lived his or her life. If a person who lived thousands of years ago made their living as a mason, their skeleton will likely show some lower back wear and the arms will have deeper grooves in the bones for larger and much-used muscles. Today the term for such things is a "repetitive stress injury." We use ergonomics to study and eventually create a better, safer work environment. Repetitive stress injury is very indicative of what is taking place—a person whose body is placed in a less than natural position repeats a particular motion thousands of times. Improper alignment of the body during *sanchin kata* can bring on or aggravate injury to, in this instance, a knee by twisting and placing improper pressure on it.

Rotating the foot

Rotating the foot outward is not done in *sanchin kata* for several reasons. Splaying the foot outward does not give the strong footing necessary. This position is simply weak. A person who stands this way can be pushed or pulled off balance quite easily. In addition, stepping forward with the foot splayed out takes the foot

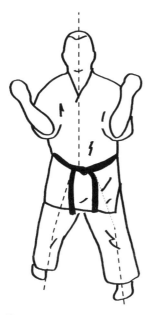

PLACEMENT OF FEET ALLOWING REFINED
BODY STRUCTURE FURTHER UP THE BODY.

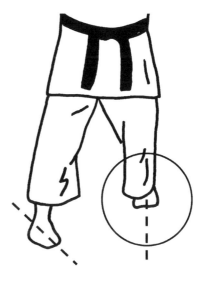

REAR FOOT SHOWING PLACEMENT OF CENTERLINE.

completely out of the movement. The rear foot when splayed outwards becomes a dead weight and the initial movement to step forward is generated in the hip, not the foot. This gross hip movement simply makes the step awkward, large, and clumsy. Conversely, rotating the foot too far inward, or in a pigeon-toed manner, goes too much the other way and again movement is generated from the hip when stepping forward.

As described earlier, the centerline of the foot is the line the rear foot uses, a very important factor for correct stepping. In nature, the higher the heel on an animal the faster it is and the longer it can sustain its speed, whereas the lower the heel the slower the animal. The lower the heel, the heavier the load it can bear. Examples of low-heeled animals include

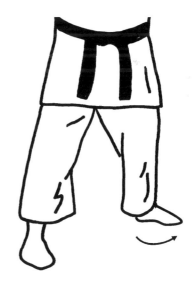

FOOT SPLAYED OUTWARD (FOOT ROTATED OUT).

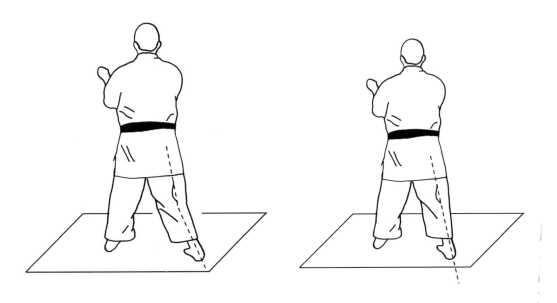

LINE FROM HEEL THROUGH CALF
SHOWING IMPROPER ALIGNMENT.

LINE FROM HEEL THROUGH CALF
SHOWING PROPER ALIGNMENT.

elephants and hippopotamuses. Although a hippopotamus can be very fast, they have difficulty sustaining their speed over long distances. The placement of the heel simply is not high enough or efficiently placed for speed over distance.

The rear foot in *sanchin kata* should be placed with the same intent as that of a high-heeled animal. By placing the rear foot on the centerline, one is able to use the calf muscle to move the foot forward and not generate movement in the hip. This results in less motion, more efficient use of stronger muscles, and increased speed.

The Feet: Test It

To do this test, you need to have someone stand in *zenkutsu dachi*, or front forward-leaning stance. This method will make the movement larger and easier to see than in *sanchin dachi*. Stand in front of your partner as if readying to fight, and have them turn the toes out on the back leg. Then ask them to kick at you with their back foot. What you will see is that the hip corresponding to the back foot will have to move first. This large movement can easily be spotted by both skilled and non-skilled martial artists. Have your partner reset their stance and place the toes forward on the back leg, which may require shortening the stance a little. Then have them kick again by lifting the heel of

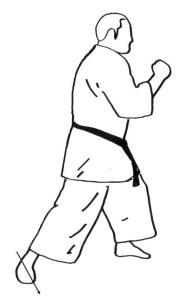

PREPARATION FOR FRONT KICK (*MAE GERI*) FROM FRONT STANCE (*ZENKUTSU DACHI*) WITH REAR FOOT TURNED OUTWARD.

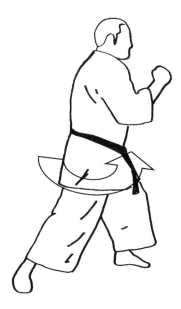

INITIAL MOVEMENT FOR KICK IS OBVIOUS BECAUSE OF LARGE HIP MOVEMENT.

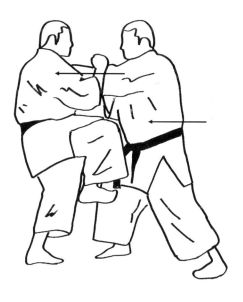

COUNTERATTACK.

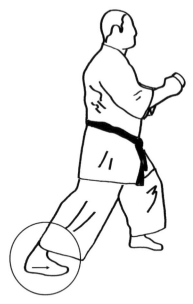

PREPARATION FOR FRONT KICK (*MAE GERI*)
FROM FRONT STANCE (*ZENKUTSU DACHI*)
WITH REAR FOOT TURNED FORWARD.

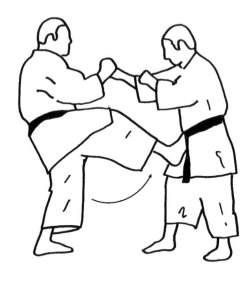

COUNTERATTACK CANNOT BE MADE.

the kicking foot first by using the calf muscle. This method makes the need for initiating hip action unnecessary and makes the kick swifter. If a kick is an over-emphasized step, then reverse engineering should make it clear that the same actions are needed for a kick in *zenkutsu dachi* and a step in *sanchin dachi*. The results are the same two items: little motion and structural integrity.

Squats are a common weightlifting activity. A weightlifter holds an iron bar behind their neck on their shoulders with weights on each end, then squats down and returns to standing. Pick up any muscle magazine or weightlifting book and you will see a constant theme that the knees should track over the toes when doing squats. The knees should not splay

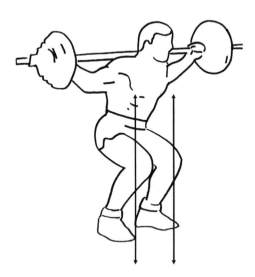

WEIGHTLIFTING EXERCISE CALLED SQUATS
WITH GOOD KNEE TRACKING.

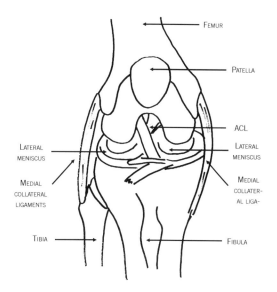

THE ANATOMY OF THE KNEE.

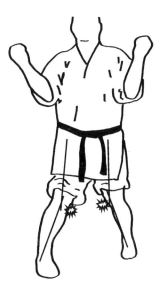

THE KNEE TRACKING INCORRECTLY TO THE INSIDE PLACING STRESS ON THE LIGAMENTS.

out nor should they collapse toward the center. Both of these are a formula for injury to the knee.

The knee should be above kidney point #1. The location is the center of the foot directly behind the two large pads that cover the ball joints of the foot. When the knee is placed at this angle, a right triangle is formed. This is important because it follows the Fibonacci Ratio.

A slight outward rotation of the knee allows the femur and tibia bones to track as nature intended, preventing undue wear on the outside contact points on the two bones. This alignment also makes a direct step forward easier because it does not involve any unnecessary motion.

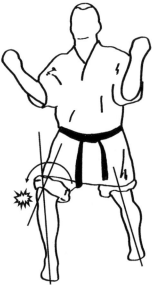

THE KNEE TRACKING INCORRECTLY TO THE
OUTSIDE PLACING STRESS ON THE LIGAMENTS

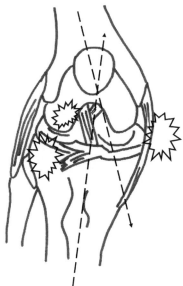

THE KNEE TRACKING INCORRECTLY.

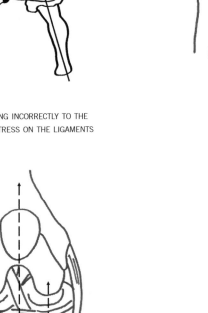

THE KNEE TRACKING CORRECTLY MAKING FOR
SMOOTH AND STRESS-FREE MOVEMENT.

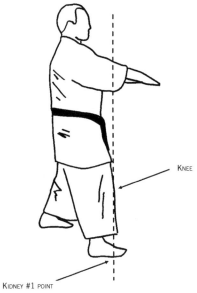

KNEE

KIDNEY #1 POINT

SIDE PICTURE OF THE KNEE CORRECTLY PLACED OVER
ACUPUNCTURE POINT KIDNEY #1 ON THE FOOT.

CHAPTER SIX

Thighs

Wealth unused might as well not exist

—*Aesop* [35]

The thighs, which are composed of the largest muscle and muscle group in the body, are a rich source of power. If one looks at the human body and tries to determine the center point, it would appear to be somewhere around the stomach area. In fact, it is located below the navel. The lungs, stomach, and large and small intestines that make up the abdomen are organs that do not possess the same density as muscle. The thighs are made up of many muscles. However, the most significant on the front of the leg is the rectus femoris sitting directly on top of the thigh, the vastus medialis on the inside of the thigh just above the knee, and its larger counterpart on the outside of the leg, the vastus lateralis. These muscles are among the most important ones for *sanchin kata*.

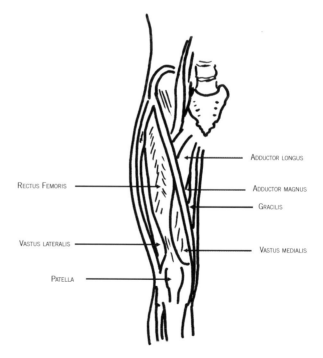

THE ANATOMY OF THE THIGH.

Labels: Rectus Femoris, Vastus lateralis, Patella, Adductor longus, Adductor magnus, Gracilis, Vastus medialis

31

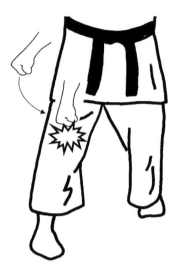

TAPPING THE TOP OF THE THIGH TO FEEL
THE TIGHTNESS OF THE MUSCLES

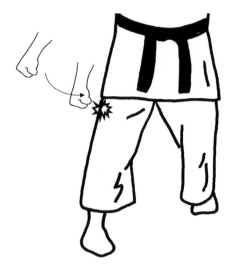

TAPPING THE SIDE OF THE THIGH TO FEEL
THE TIGHTNESS OF THE MUSCLES.

Thighs: Test It

Standing in *sanchin dachi* with your same arm as your lead leg, reach down and poke the top of your thigh with your index finger. It should be firm but not hard. Now reach around the outside of your lead thigh, the vastus lateralis, and, using your finger, again poke your thigh. The difference in intensity should be great. The top of the thigh will remain firm but not tight while in *sanchin dachi* and the outside of the thigh, the vastus lateralis will be strong, firm, and tight.

CHAPTER SEVEN

Hips

Moto, Moto, Moto
(Translation: More, More, More)

—*Judo Sensei to his student as he turns*
his hips in preparation of a throw. [36]

The hips are to be square to the form. If a person is facing a wall while doing *sanchin kata,* the hips should remain square to the wall. When stepping, it is important to be attentive to not leaving a hip behind. As one steps forward, oftentimes the hip that does not move gets left behind and is brought forward after the fact, and set after the stepping has finished. Even slightly doing this delays the setting of the technique and disrupts the architecture of the form. There is a tendency among some practitioners to leave the side of the hip with the rear leg slightly back while standing still. Standing with one hip back should be avoided because it makes the stance weak, requires the hip to be moved prior to the leg, and segments the body, not all of which are advantageous to swift, powerful movement.

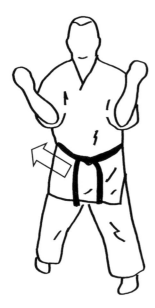

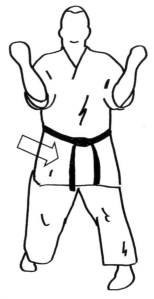

FACING IN *SANCHIN DACHI* WITH THE REAR HIP HELD BACK.

FACING IN *SANCHIN DACHI* WITH THE REAR HIP HELD FORWARD IN PROPER ALIGNMENT.

Hips: Test It

Stand in front of a mirror in *sanchin dachi,* let one side of your hip fall, or slip back a little. This position takes less effort and opens up the hips. Now step forward while watching yourself in the mirror. You will find that a large movement originates in the hip. The reason for this gross movement is that the hip needs to travel further and it needs to move first prior to the step. Opening the hip, or having the hips twisted so one is back of the other creates a bigger *ski*. A larger *ski*, or opening is not desirable because it makes the practitioner more vulnerable. Now reset your position and this time twist the hip on the rear leg side forward bringing the hip square to the mirror. Again, step and notice as the hips and the body move as one unit. This unified movement gains the practitioner structural integrity and speed because all parts move as a single unit.

CHAPTER EIGHT

The Trunk of a Strong Tree

In union there is strength.

—*Aesop* [37]

The sacrum is a bone shaped like an inverted triangle that sits at the end of the lumbar region. The sacrum also forms the back of the pelvic girdle. To make the spine as straight as possible, it is necessary to tilt the sacrum. When a person is straightening their spine, it can appear the person is thrusting their hips forward. Because the sacrum is attached to the rest to the pelvic girdle including the hipbones, when the sacrum is straightened into a vertical alignment, the whole pelvic girdle moves forward, giving the illusion the hips are the key to correct position of the pelvic girdle. The fact is the hips are not the object of attention but merely an indicator of the sacrum being in the correct position. Oftentimes a thrusting of the pelvis forward on the step is done by the practitioner of *sanchin kata* to the extent that the *obi*, or belt, actually does a little flip from the thrust. While this is a good training aid for the beginner, for the more skilled practitioner it is an unnecessary overemphasis. This kind of thrust is actually an attempt to move the sacrum at the base of the spine to align with the spinal column as needed for the correct posture for *sanchin kata*. The tucking under of the pelvis and the little flip of the *obi* put the mind in the front of the body when it should be focused on the sacrum and downward, not up and out.

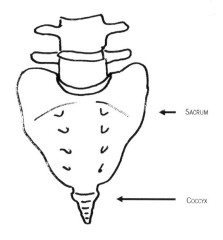

THE ANATOMY OF THE SACRUM.

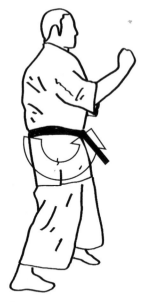

BELT FLIP SEEN FROM THE SIDE.

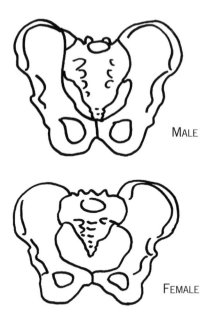

MALE

FEMALE

THE PELVIC GIRDLE.

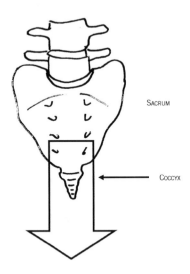

SACRUM

COCCYX

PELVIS HELD VERTICAL BY PULLING THE COCCYX DOWN
STRAIGHTENING THE SACRUM.

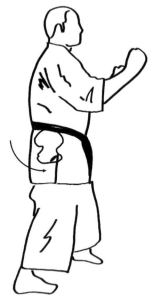

PELVIS TUCKED UNDERNEATH. VIEW FROM THE SIDE.

CHAPTER NINE

 # Movement Not Seen

When you decide to attack, keep calm and dash in quickly, forestalling the enemy.

—*Miyamoto Musashi* [38]

The Parallax

Parallax is a word common to astronomy; it is also called triangulation. Parallax allows astronomers to judge distance or a military radio operator to find another radio. In nature, it allows predators to judge the distance to their meal. As a rule, a predator has their eyes in the front of their head for stereoscopic forward vision that allows for triangulation. To provide peripheral vision, predators turn their heads.

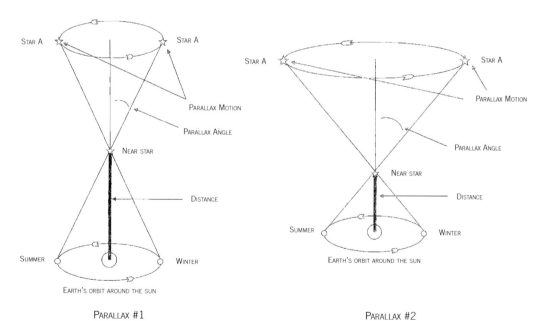

PARALLAX #1   PARALLAX #2

Herbivores have their eyes on the sides of their heads giving them a much wider vision, yet they cannot see well directly in front of themselves. When a bird tries to look closely at something on the ground, they turn their head and place one eye on the subject. Each form of eye placement has an inherent advantage and disadvantage. Humans, who like predators, have front-set eyes, use parallax to judge distance.

Simply put, given three points, one can judge their distance from an object. The first two points, in this instance would be the eyes, the left eye being the first point, and the right eye the second point. The third point of the triangulation would be the object at which one is looking. Naturally, using this information, one is able to judge distance because of the movement of the background.

Movement: Test It 1

Hold your thumb up at arm's length and look at a wall with just one eye. Then close that eye and look at your thumb with your other eye. Your thumb will seem to shift its position against the wall. Viewing an object from two different perspectives makes it to seem to move between two positions, at least compared to its background.

Now move your thumb closer to your face and repeat looking at the wall with each eye. The shift of your thumb will be greater. The closer the object the larger the shift allowing you to judge distance in the same way the astronomer does when looking at the stars.

Another example of this parallax shift occurs while sitting in a moving car and watching a fence go by. The fence close to the road moves quite quickly, whereas the house set back from the road moves more slowly. This is one reason that *sanchin kata* does not cock a punch by pulling the hand back to get power as in a Hollywood movie. The pulling back, or cocking, of the hand gives the opponent an opportunity to see the strike coming, find the strike in space, and judge the distance and the momentum. Cocking the punch in the classic chamber position makes the parallax shift more difficult to detect by making it more acute. As the star viewed in the parallax shift part of the illustration, the star in the background that is used to judge the distance has a very small shift. In a situation where a strike is a surprise, the opponent is unable to judge the distance or speed and their amygdala, sometimes called the lizard brain, brain goes into flight reflex.

Think of the owl shifting its head back and forth multiple times while it judges its prey from a tree limb. The owl is augmenting its natural forward eye parallax with several other positions all designed to get a better judgment on the distance of its next meal. Humans do the same thing. For example, a person driving in snow, rain, and fog or having a hard time seeing what is taking place up the road—maybe an accident has happened. In this situation, one will naturally do what the owl does,

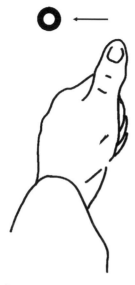

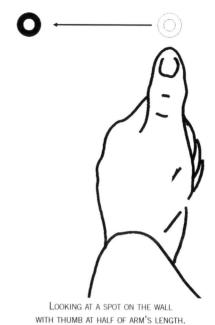

LOOKING AT A SPOT ON THE WALL
WITH THUMB AT ARM'S LENGTH.

LOOKING AT A SPOT ON THE WALL
WITH THUMB AT HALF OF ARM'S LENGTH.

crane the neck up, down, and side to side in an effort to get as much information about how far away your subject of focus is from you. This is a natural and instinctual behavior that humans often do unconsciously.

Movement: Test It 2

An excellent way to demonstrate this shift is to take a *bo* and swing it like a baseball bat toward the head of a person. The person who is having the *bo* swung at them will easily be able to discern the timing of the swing and lift their arm to block the swinging *bo* with confidence. Now hold the *bo* with the tip pointed at the face of the other person. While sliding the *bo* through the lead hand, thrust the tip of the *bo* to their face. The swifter you move and the less motion you make, the more the other person's reaction will be to flinch away from the thrusting tip.

In the first scenario, the *bo* swinging from the side allows the upper brain to be active and wrest control from the amygdala, or lizard brain. In the second example, the lizard brain is engaged in deciding two actions—fight or flight—due to the lack of a parallax shift. This lack of shift means decisions need to be made instantly. Oftentimes, the decision made is to retreat, to accumulate more information.

When we move in *sanchin kata,* our goal is to deny our opponent the ability to use parallax shift to gauge distance or speed, or both. The second part of the action

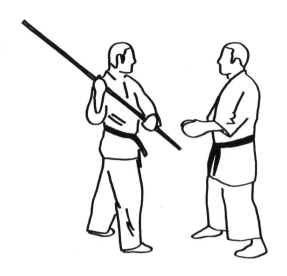

PREPARING *BO* SWING TO SIDE OF HEAD.

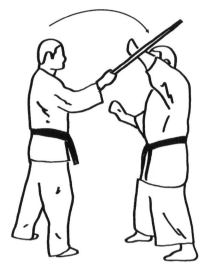

SWINGING *BO* AT SIDE OF HEAD WITH BLOCK RESPONSE.

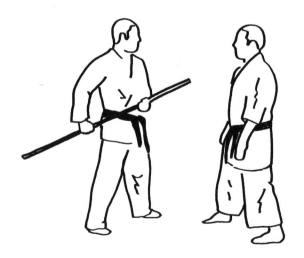

PREPARING *BO* THRUST TO FACE.

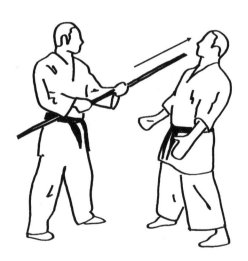

THRUSTING *BO* TO FACE WITH RECOIL REACTION.

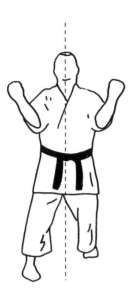

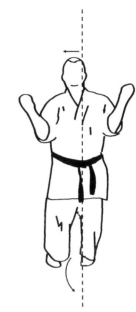

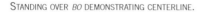

STANDING OVER *BO* DEMONSTRATING CENTERLINE.

WALKING WITH OVEREMPHASIS ON THE CRESCENT STEP DEMONSTRATING SIDE-TO-SIDE WOBBLE.

of denying them this ability is that the lizard brain takes over and you elicit a flinch reaction from the opponent as they react to the incoming threat. This flinch reaction can be as large as leaning back and lifting the arms to a simple "brain burp" as they control their flinch reaction and the higher brain audits the moment's events. The flinch reaction can be trained out of a person but is very difficult to do because it requires the mind to override the basic fight-or-flight instinct. This is the moment of advantage, the opening, or the *ski* in Japanese.

CHAPTER TEN

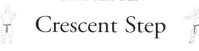

Crescent Step

Sometimes a cigar is just a cigar.

—*Sigmund Freud*[39]

The *crescent step* is used in stepping in *sanchin kata*. It is called a crescent step because the path that the advancing foot traces on the floor resembles a crescent moon. Overthinking the crescent step can cause a practitioner to spend too much effort on a movement that is fundamental and simple at the same time. Often the focus is on the step and the feet, and, although this is important, this focus places the emphasis on the end of the action and not the root movement. When the focus is placed on the end action, the fundamentals can be lost and the crescent step is no exception. In an effort to deny the opponent the opportunity to detect parallax shift via any extraneous movement or to give them a cue to your actions, it is important to make no lateral movement. When executing the crescent step, the action is direct-ed forward to the opponent and not to the sides.

There is a distinct difference between walking and the kind of stepping one does in *sanchin kata*. A walk is a controlled fall. That is to say that for a moment, when walking, one is literally falling a short distance. One balances on one foot for a moment and leans forward as the other foot is picked up and placed in front. For that brief moment, one has moved from being balanced on one foot to shifting their weight forward and falling onto their other foot. Stepping in *sanchin kata* is differ-ent from walking in that the first motion of the step is not to shift the weight to one leg like in walking, but to move forward by bending the forward knee and pulling with the lead foot. In this manner, the practitioner moves forward not sideways, which avoids a parallax shift and controls their balance by having the moving foot remain in contact with the ground.

The difference between *sanchin kata* stepping and natural stepping is shown in the graph below. While not scientific, the graph is useful as an illustration of the loss of power in walking. Walking, because it is a controlled fall, is based more on gravi-ty than muscular power. *Sanchin kata* stepping is based on muscular power and less in gravity. The first illustration shows the power line dipping severely while the per-

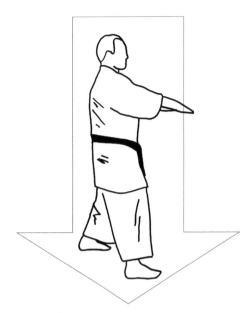

SANCHIN DACHI STEPPING PREPARATION.

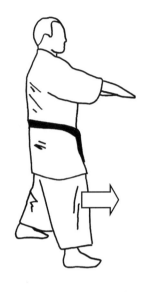

SANCHIN DACHI STEPPING WITH
INITIAL FORWARD KNEE MOVEMENT.

son is balanced on one foot and preparing to fall into the next step. This weakness comes first from the falling involved in the stepping action and secondly from the rear foot first orientation. A lean of the upper body is required to un-weight the rear foot. During *sanchin kata* stepping, the power line stays straight. This is because the initial stepping action is one of pulling with the front foot so the body does not lean and stays vertical and balanced.

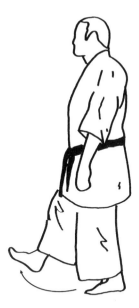

STAGE 1. WALKING USES A CONTROLLED FALL. LITERALLY BALANCING ON ONE FOOT AND FALLING ONTO THE OTHER.

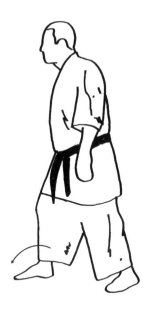

STAGE 2. COMPLETION OF WALKING CONTROLLED FALL.

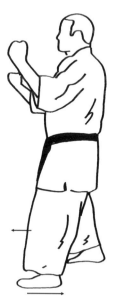

STAGE 1 *SANCHIN KATA* STEPPING BEGINNING POSITION WITH INITIAL MOTION OF FORWARD FOOT PULL.

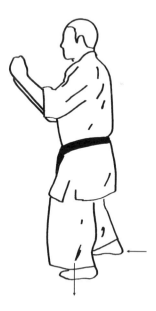

STAGE 2. COMPLETION OF *SANCHIN KATA* STEPPING.

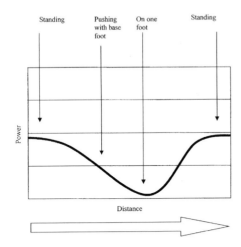

POWER GRAPH: WALKING.

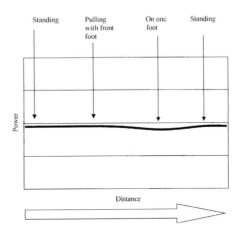

POWER GRAPH: *SANCHIN KATA* STEPPING.

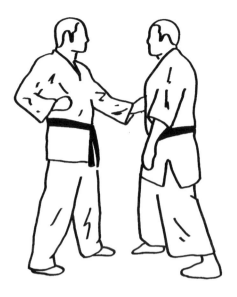
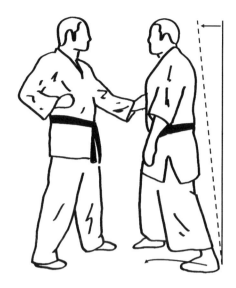

PARTNERS BEGIN FACING EACH OTHER WITH THE TESTER PLACING A VERTICAL FIST ON THE CHEST OF THE PERSON WHO IS HAVING THEIR CRESCENT (*SANCHIN KATA*) STEP TESTED.

ATTEMPT TO "WALK" INTO THE TESTER'S FIST.

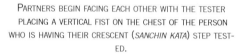

Crescent Step: Test It 1

After your partner places a vertical fist on your chest giving pressure, attempt to walk into the fist. You will not be able to move forward because you have leaned into the fist and are trying a controlled fall, a walk. Stop and reset the test. Now this time, step with *sanchin kata* stepping, pulling with the front foot instead of walking as you did before. You will move forward easily.

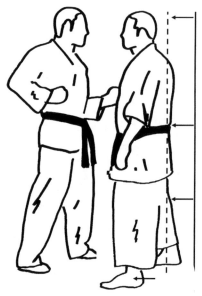

PARTNERS BEGIN FACING EACH OTHER WITH THE TESTER
PLACING A VERTICAL FIST TESTING *SANCHIN KATA*.

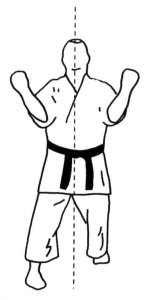

FACING MIRROR STANDING OVER A *BO*.

Crescent Step: Test It 2

Stand in front of a mirror, the larger the better. Using tape, make a straight line on the floor or have somebody else watch you step forward in *sanchin dachi*. If your first move was to lean to one side, putting all your weight on one leg, you are not moving toward your target. To lean to one side and then the other as you step is a waste of motion and of time. To remove this lean, bend with the lead leg at the knee making your first motion a forward motion. Then let the other leg draw up naturally and in a crescent step pass the other foot on its way to the next position. This method makes all motions go forward and reduces side-to-side leaning to a minimum.

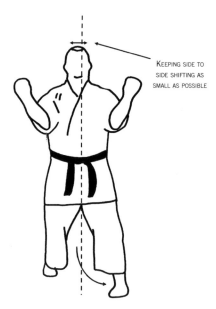

KEEPING SIDE TO
SIDE SHIFTING AS
SMALL AS POSSIBLE

FACING MIRROR AND STEPPING FORWARD
WHILE NOT SHIFTING FROM SIDE TO SIDE.

CHAPTER ELEVEN

The Spine

One thousand days to learn; ten thousand days to refine.

—*Japanese Proverb*

The spine, the vertebral column, or the backbone, which is part of the axial (upper body) skeleton, forms a strong but flexible shaft that supports the upper body, the ribcage, shoulders, and head. Because of its flexibility, the spine needs support, which is provided by ligaments and muscle. It also houses the spinal cord, the neurological highway of communication between the brain and the rest of the body. The intervertebral discs or simply, disks, serve the role of the body's shock absorbers, protecting the vertebrae, brain, and other structures. The bones of the spine are grouped into three major sets: the cervical vertebrae, the thoracic vertebrae, the lumbar vertebrae, the sacrum (five fused vertebrae) and the coccyx (four fused vertebrae). For our purposes, we will discuss the last two sets of fused vertebrae as the sacrum and the coccyx and the other three sets by individual numbers in descending order from the base of the skull.

The cervical vertebrae are numbered one through seven starting at the base of the skull.

The next set are the thoracic vertebrae, composed of twelve vertebrae, then the final set of non-fused vertebrae, the lumbar, composed of five. These three sets make a total of twenty-four non-fused vertebrae.

Curvature

Each one of the three sets of vertebrae has a curvature moving front to back. Curvature from side to side causes problems on many levels. One well-known condition of this kind is scoliosis, a chronic form of lateral side-to-side curvature. The seven cervical vertebrae have a curve toward the front of the body at the throat. The next twelve vertebrae, the thoracic, curve the other way away from the solar plexus. The last five, the lumbar curve back to the center of the body, moving into the body. The most acute curves are in the fused vertebrae the sacrum and the coccyx, which curve in the opposite direction of each other, forming the sacral curvature.[40]

The practice of *sanchin kata* straightens the spine taking some of the natural curvature of the spine away. In many schools when the basics of *sanchin kata* are taught, one of the techniques is to tell the student to pull their buttocks together tightly. This action forces the lower part of the sacrum forward giving it the desired vertical position. This can create issues later in the practice of the *kata* because the overly tight buttocks restrict a free-flowing stepping ability. By pushing the pelvis forward too much, a domino effect of undesirable results is created. This negative effect can be seen most easily in the abdominal area. When the buttock is pinched together and drawn underneath, the pelvis is rocked upward and the sternum, or breastbone, is dropped forward, shortening the stomach area. When the pelvis is rolled forward, and the sternum is rolled forward and down in an attempt to shorten and create muscular tension in the abdomen, the diaphragm is restricted. A restricted diaphragm is similar to a birdcage. If you put a balloon in a birdcage and blow up

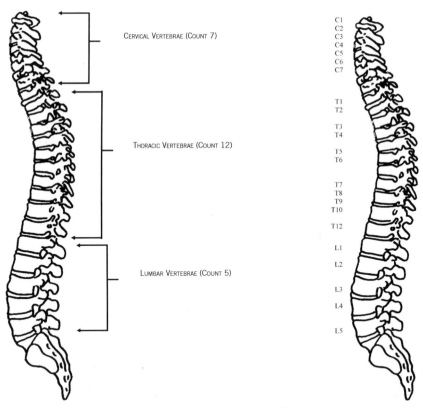

SPINE ANNOTATED WITH NAMES OF SECTIONS.   SPINE ANNOTATED WITH NUMBERS OF VERTEBRAE.

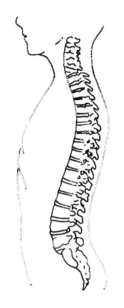

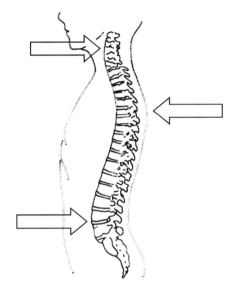

SPINE WITH NATURAL CURVE.   SPINE WITH CURVE REMOVED.

the balloon, it only has so much room in which to expand. This version of the bird-cage is similar to the case of a pelvis rocked forward and the sternum pulled down. The expansion of the lungs or balloon is restricted by the ribs, or birdcage. Removing the bottom of the birdcage allows for the expansion of the balloon downward unrestricted. Continuing the analogy, the lungs, with the bottom of the birdcage removed are then limited only by the movement of the diaphragm. The diaphragm is in turn restricted by its range of movement and other physical restrictions. When keeping the proper structure in the alignment of the sacrum, the stomach is opened up allowing the diaphragm the greatest freedom of movement.

A second feature resulting from the pinching of the pelvis and sternum together is the shoving of the entrails up in the abdominal cavity thus reducing the room in the stomach area. This shoving of the entrails upward also restricts the ability of the diaphragm to move freely and expand downward, decreasing inhalation capacity.

The Coccyx

To achieve the proper alignment of the sacrum, it is important to focus on an even smaller part of the body, the coccyx, commonly called the tailbone. Pointing the coccyx downward the sacrum becomes more vertical without creating a problem higher up and in the abdomen as previously mentioned. It is not necessary to thrust the sacrum down or the pelvis forward. Simply moving the sacrum into as much of a vertical position as is needed to form the alignments further up the spine is all that

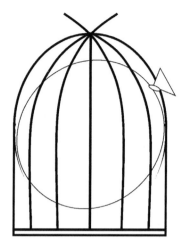

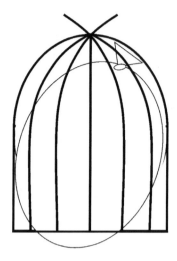

BIRDCAGE AND BALLOON ANALOGY
SHOWING RESTRICTED BREATHING.

BIRDCAGE AND BALLOON ANALOGY
SHOWING ROOM FOR MORE BREATH.

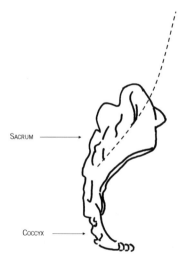

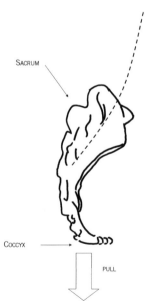

COCCYX TILT IN NATURAL POSITION.

COCCYX TILT IN SANCHIN KATA POSITION.

is required. When focusing on the coccyx, the placement of the entire pelvic girdle achieves the necessary natural balance and the proper alignment without affectation and exaggeration.

Thoracic Vertebra Number Eleven

As already pointed out, the beginning of this process of straightening begins with the coccyx and sacrum, and moves up the spine to the vertebra called thoracic number eleven (T-11). It can also be found a little more easily by counting up seven vertebrae from the sacrum. T-11 is significant in that the diaphragm makes contact in this region. The spine at T-11 serves as the point of origin for the diaphragm. *Sanchin kata* requires the spine's natural curvature to be countered here at T-11, pushing this vertebra opposite, or backward, from the way it normally rests.

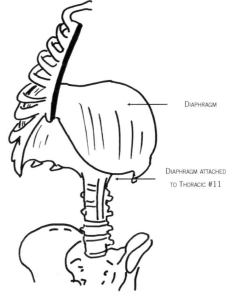

DIAPHRAGM

DIAPHRAGM ATTACHED
TO THORACIC #11

DIAPHRAGM WITH CONNECTION TO THORACIC
VERTEBRA NUMBER ELEVEN (T-11).

The Spine: Test It 1

One way to begin to experience this is to stand against a wall and place the back of your pelvis and your shoulder blades against the wall. Slowly start to straighten your lower back trying to touch the wall with the lower curve of your back. It is difficult if not impossible for many people to keep their sacrum in a vertical position and push T-11 back so far as to touch the wall as well. The key here is balance, moving T-11 as close as possible to touching the wall while also keeping the sacrum vertical. Because each person is unique, the essence of this exercise is for you to gain insight as to how your spine feels when these come into alignment. Once you are able to feel the alignment and begin to become familiar with it, feel free to move away from the wall and attempt to gain the same sensation of having this alignment without the support of the wall.

Next, cervical vertebra number seven (C-7) needs to be brought into line with the sacrum and the T-11. C-7 is located seven vertebrae below the base of the skull. To bring this into line with the coccyx, sacrum, and T-11 is a far different process than the previous actions. To begin, it is important to have the lower parts of the spine already in place. Standing straight, use your chest muscles to bring the shoul-

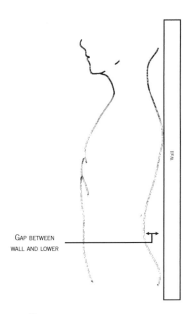

GAP BETWEEN
WALL AND LOWER

PLACING BACK AGAINST WALL SHOWING
GAP BETWEEN WALL AND SPINE.

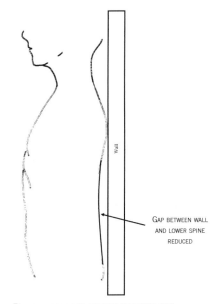

GAP BETWEEN WALL
AND LOWER SPINE
REDUCED

PLACING THE BACK AGAINST THE WALL AND
REMOVING THE GAP BETWEEN WALL AND SPINE.

ders slightly forward of the center of the midway point of the torso. The shoulders-back military attention chest posture during *sanchin kata* should be avoided. Holding the shoulders back can create incidental lifting of the shoulders toward the ears, creating a position of tension that is not beneficial. Instead, a natural position is achieved by letting the shoulder relax to their normal resting position. The shoulders now set, naturally in the front half of the torso body, do not split the difference between the front of the body. Pulling the shoulder too far forward can cause a caved-in chest. The practitioner needs to be mindful to avoid this collapsed chest position. This chest position also closes, but does not cave. It is important to note here that when breathing the chest and shoulders should not move.

Cervical Vertebra Number One

Working on the back of the head is the next step to ensure that the spine is in the correct alignment. By pulling the back of the head backward and over the spine, the chin is pulled in. In many traditional methods of instruction, the chin is emphasized because it is the fastest means of putting the skull into the right position. Often when a person is asked to move their head backward to align the top part of the spine, a person will tilt their head backward. So to avoid this natural reaction, the chin is emphasized. This means of instruction is actually about the back of the head, not the chin and is not to protect the throat as often said. No advantage in protecting the throat is gained by pulling the chin in. The body when under stress or preparing for conflict protects the throat by rotating the head downward, exposing the front skull, and reducing the exposure of the throat. This motion is called, "bowing the neck." This bowing of the neck is a common body preparation prior to attack. People skilled in violence will use bowing of the neck as an indicator of imminent attack.

Pulling the chin too far into the throat is actually detrimental to the structure of the form because it restricts breathing and places undue emphasis on constriction of breathing that result in a harsh raspy sound as if the practitioner is clearing their throat.

The goal of pulling the chin backward toward the throat is to place the skull over cervical vertebra number one (C1), at the very top of the spine without rolling the head backward.

The Spine: Test It 2

Stand in the opening movement of *sanchin kata* with double chest blocks (*morote kamae*). Have your partner place a vertical fist at the top of your sternum. Slide your chin slightly forward, just a fin-

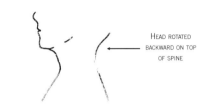

HEAD ROTATED BACKWARD ON TOP OF SPINE

HEAD RIDING NATURALLY ON TOP OF SPINE.

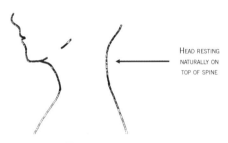

HEAD RESTING NATURALLY ON TOP OF SPINE

HEAD TILTED BACKWARD.

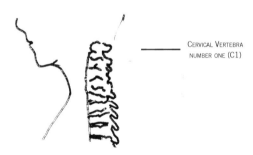

CERVICAL VERTEBRA NUMBER ONE (C1)

HEAD POSITION AFTER CERVICAL VERTEBRA NUMBER ONE (C1) IS PULLED INTO *SANCHIN KATA* POSITION.

ger width, or two. Then have your partner press their fist into your sternum in an attempt to push you back. After feeling the experience, reset yourself into the same position and this time move the C1 at the base of your skull back and over the rest of your spine. It is important to keep your jaw line level. Rocking the head is detrimental to *sanchin kata* and this test as well. With your head and C1 in place, your partner now presses into your sternum with their fist in an attempt to push you off your base. You will feel a distinct difference in the amount of pressure you are able

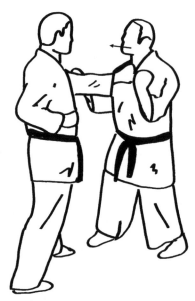

MOROTE KAMAE WITH VERTICAL FIST GIVING
PRESSURE ON CHEST WITH CHIN FORWARD.

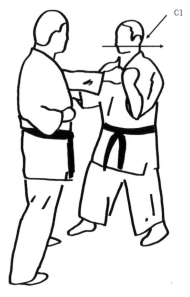

MOROTE KAMAE WITH VERTICAL FIST GIVING PRESSURE
ON CHEST WITH C1 PULLED INTO PLACE, PULLING THE
CHIN BACKWARD.

to withstand. Experiment with different positions and you will find that the correct position for *sanchin kata*, chin down and C1 pulled back offer the strongest position.

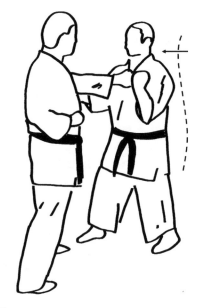

C1 IN *SANCHIN KATA* POSITION MAKES STANCE STRONGER.

CHAPTER TWELVE

Shoulders

I will master something, then the creativity will come.

—Japanese Proverb

The shoulders should sit naturally on top of the ribcage slightly forward. During most of the day, we roll our shoulders forward caving in the chest to varying degrees. Some people roll their shoulders so far forward they create an arched back in combination with a caved chest. These are excellent examples of precisely what you do not want to do.

Again, to emphasize this unnatural combination of rolling the shoulders slightly forward, yet still lifting the clavicles or collarbones and dropping the sternum is very important. Be mindful not to roll the sternum forward, resulting in the top of the sternum being forward of the bottom of the sternum, because this causes the chest to cave inward and a hunching of the back. Instead, pull the sternum down, keeping it vertical. Again, this is about locking in the bones via muscle tension in an unusual position. It takes practice to avoid hunching the back while crunching the chest down and closing the solar plexus.

Shoulders: Test It

The most basic form of testing the *sanchin dachi* stance is to simply press into the sternum, the chest, of a person who has rolled their shoulders too far forward. The instability of their stance is easy to see and their balance can be displaced with little effort.

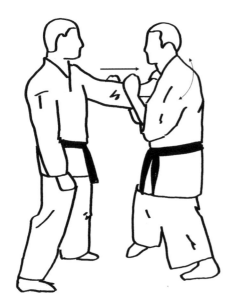

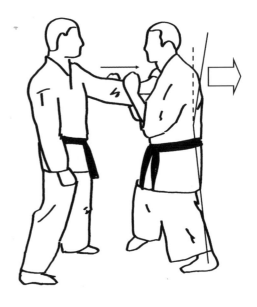

MOROTE KAMAE WITH VERTICAL FIST GIVING PRESSURE ON
CHEST WITH SHOULDERS ROLLED TOO FAR FORWARD.

SHOULDERS ROLLED FORWARD RESULTS IN
BROKEN STANCE, PUSHED OFF BALANCE.

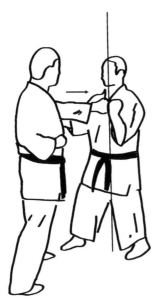

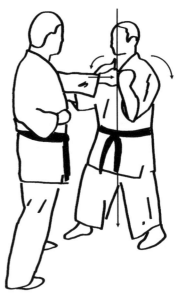

MOROTE KAMAE WITH VERTICAL FIST GIVING PRESSURE ON
CHEST WITH SHOULDERS HELD FORWARD SLIGHTLY AND
DOWNWARD IN *SANCHIN KATA* POSITION.

SANCHIN KATA POSITION WITH SHOULDER HELD
SLIGHTLY FORWARD AND IN DOWN POSITION RESULTS
IN STRONGER STANCE.

CHAPTER THIRTEEN

Arms

*Coming together is a beginning, staying together
is progress, and working together is success.*

—*Henry Ford* [41]

The point of origin of the arm is the shoulder. The shoulder is an inherently unstable ball joint dangling from the side of the chest. The shoulder trades stability for mobility as the support for the joint comes from muscles. The largest muscles holding the joint in place are the pectoralis major and minor, the latissimus dorsi, and the deltoid muscle.

Understanding the interplay of these muscles is important to executing a powerful *sanchin kata*. As noted in Chapter Four, in Traditional Chinese Medicine as well as in martial arts including *Tai Chi Chuan* and karate, the measurement of a *kua*, which is equal to the size of an individual's fist, is used. The measurement is used to determine the proper distance of the elbow from the rib cage. This distance allows a person to tighten their pectoral and latissimus muscles, holding the deltoid firm but unflexed. By reaching across one's body and pressing into the deltoid muscle, one should be able to feel it in a relaxed state. By lifting the elbow out from the body slightly, one should be able to feel the deltoid muscle contract. This contraction of the deltoid muscle is not correct because it slows down the strike. The tightening of the deltoid indicates that the first motion of the strike is not directed forward toward the target, but instead is directed laterally away from the striker's own body. In addition, the tightening increases the time it takes to strike as the

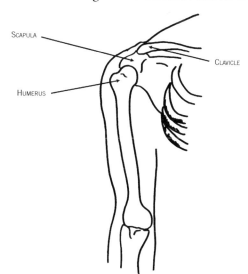

ANATOMY OF THE SHOULDER.

motion becomes larger. By tightening the pectoral and latissimus muscles, the shoulder is stabilized. The deltoid muscle is removed from the process, speed is increased, and finally, the strike is directed at the target in the most expedient way, relaxed and swift.

Upon impact of the strike, the bicep and triceps as well as the forearm muscles, should snap into full tension upon complete extension, and then relax to a toned readiness.

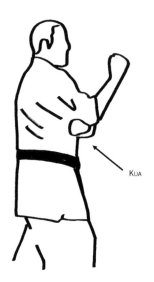

DEMONSTRATING THE CORRECT DISTANCE (ONE *KUA*)
OF BLOCKING ELBOW FROM RIBCAGE.

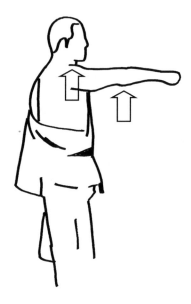

STRAIGHT CHEST PUNCH FORWARD WITH SLIGHT ELBOW LIFT
TIGHTENING THE DELTOID (SHOULDER) MUSCLE.

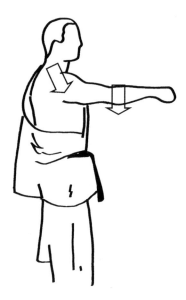

STRAIGHT CHEST PUNCH FORWARD WITH NO ELBOW LIFT
TIGHTENING THE DELTOID (SHOULDER) MUSCLE.

CHAPTER FOURTEEN

The Fist

When pure knuckles meet pure flesh, that's pure Karate,
no matter who executes it or whatever style is involved

— *Ed Parker* [42]

Some versions of *sanchin kata* use a rotating fist and others an open hand. These versions do not challenge the core essentials of the form and in some instances provide more color and variety, allowing a student to choose what system best suits their needs. If a system uses open hands or *nukite,* then that is what should be done, if a closed rotating fist, then that is what should be done. The rotation of the fist follows the Fibonacci Ratio as well. The fist does not begin the rotation from palm up to palm down until the fist enters into the second section of the ratio.

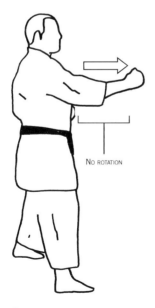

CHEST PUNCH HOLDING ROTATION.

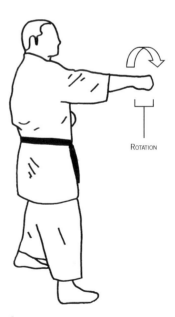

CHEST PUNCH SHOWING FINAL ROTATION
IN LAST PART OF FIBONACCI RATIO.

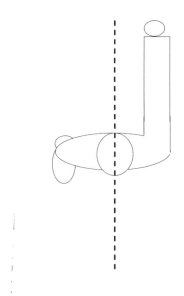

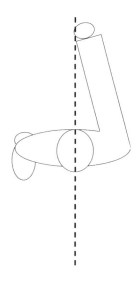

OVERHEAD VIEW OF STRIKING ARM NINETY DEGREES TO BODY.

OVERHEAD VIEW OF STRIKING ARM MOVING DOWN CENTERLINE OF BODY.

This twisting in the second section of the ratio allows for a greater snap. More importantly, this rotation point prevents the elbow from flying out from the body, keeping the path of the fist linear and the arm structurally sound for the duration of the motion. The fist should come out from the shoulder to a person's centerline. This allows one to generate power via body mass as well as to tighten the pectoral muscle, giving support to the shoulder as discussed earlier. Just as the elbow should not be bent at contact, because it becomes a shock absorber, nor should the shoulder move.

Creating a ninety-degree angle between the chest and the arm allows the body to twist away from the strike upon impact. This ninety-degree chest-to-shoulder angle is not preferred—not only because of the already mentioned impact twist, but also because it does not allow for the use of the muscles in their strongest manner. By watching a serious weightlifter working with free weights, one can see the use of the contracted pectoral muscle. Using dumbbells, a weightlifter lies down on his back and begins a "fly" by moving the dumbbells from a spread-wide position to vertical in front of their chest. This last position, vertical, allows the pectoral muscle to be contracted to its maximum amount. This is similar to the final position of a chest punch or *chudan tsuki*. The shoulder comes forward from the tension of the pectoral muscle and should not move forward any more than is necessary to tighten the mus-

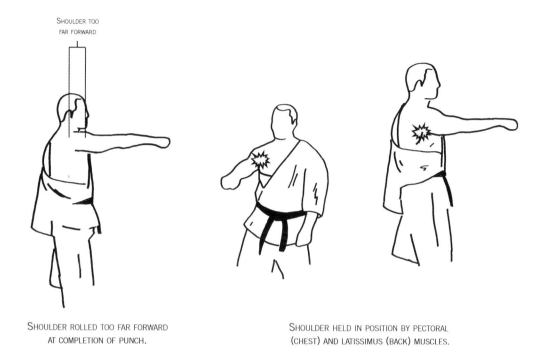

SHOULDER TOO
FAR FORWARD

SHOULDER ROLLED TOO FAR FORWARD
AT COMPLETION OF PUNCH.

SHOULDER HELD IN POSITION BY PECTORAL
(CHEST) AND LATISSIMUS (BACK) MUSCLES.

cle and anchor the shoulder. Any more forward movement weakens the position of the latissimus muscles.

To roll the shoulder too far forward creates imbalance by placing too much weight forward and causes a person to be in a leaning, thus vulnerable, position.

The Fist: Test It 1

This can be tested by grabbing the wrist directly behind the fist with two fingers. You will find it easy to unbalance the striker with little effort. A severely hunched back conspires to create a weak spine at the area between the scapulae, or the shoulder blades. This also pushes the chin forward, which, as already discussed, is a poor structural position. Have your partner then reset the shoulder into the ninety-degree position as described above and attempt with the same grip to try to pull the striker. The result will be very different.

When retracting the striking hand, the same Fibonacci Ratio applies here as well. When pulling back, it is important that the hand be held in the striking position for the first inch or so during retraction. Just prior to contact when punching, the hand completes the rotation. This position is repeated in reverse as you retract the hand. This movement can often be overlooked. After the initial pull, the rotation then begins and not before. The elbow of the arm then rests against the first attached rib.

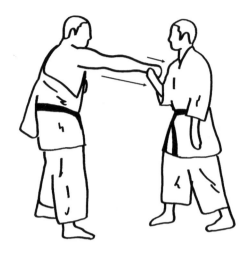

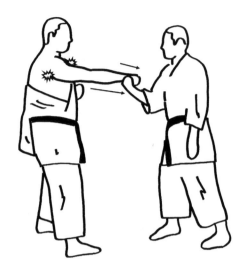

SHOULDER ROLLED TOO FAR FORWARD AT COMPLETION OF PUNCH AND USING TWO FINGERS TO PULL STRIKER OFF BALANCE.

SHOULDER HELD IN POSITION BY PECTORAL (CHEST) AND LATISSIMUS (BACK) MUSCLES ATTEMPTING MOVEMENT WITH TWO FINGERS.

The Fist: Test It 2

To demonstrate the reason for this action is to omit the punch out and having your training partner grab your wrist. Without pulling the little inch or so, try to rotate your arm into the *chudan uke* position or the chest block; it is difficult but achievable.

Now repeat the test with a slight pull first, and then with the rotation to the *chudan uke* position. The second one is easier because you have used *kuzushi*, or imbalance. This *kuzushi* breaks the other person's position on the ground and allows you to pull them into a very favorable position for you and a very poor one for them.

The Fist: Test It 3

The first punch of the *kata* takes place in *sanchin dachi* stance. Have your partner place their open hand over your punching fist while still in chamber. Move your punching fist ahead about one fist distance (*kua*) from chamber, and then rotate your fist completely over so that your fist is palm down and the thumb is toward your body. Now have your partner give enough pressure to your punching fist to slow it to a stop. At this point, it is rare that you will not splay your elbow outward away from your body to compensate for the pressure. Moving your elbow outward sets off a series of events that destroys the integrity and the power of your strike as a result

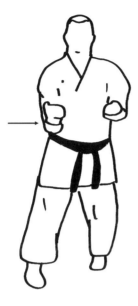

ELBOW ATTACHED TO RIBS DURING
PUNCHING PROCESS.

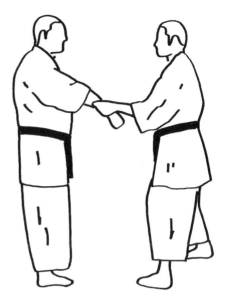

GRIPPING WRIST AND ATTEMPTING TO MOVE TO CHEST BLOCK
POSITION USING SWEEPING MOTION AS INITIAL MOVEMENT.

of moving the energy of the strike outward and not toward the target. When the elbow splays outward, the power and weight of the entire body is lost. To compensate for this loss, the deltoid muscle is activated, making your strike slower than it should be.

Repeat the same test, but this time keep the elbow in next to your body and the fist palm up until the elbow passes the ribs. This technique in combination with a solid stance should result in a strong punch that will withstand the test of your partner's pressure as they try to stop your punch.

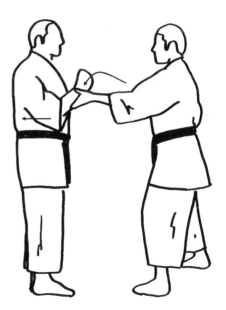

GRIPPING WRIST AND ATTEMPTING TO MOVE TO CHEST BLOCK
POSITION USING PULLING MOTION AS INITIAL MOVEMENT.

CHAPTER FIFTEEN

Knuckles

A pint of sweat saves a gallon of blood.

—*George S. Patton* [43]

Our two hands alone contain one-quarter of the bones of the adult human. They are able to perform a broad range of tasks, from removing a sliver from a child's hand to smashing boards. The hands are a means of communication, with simple gestures to full-blown languages. They communicate a range of emotions from anger to love.

The striking surface of the *seiken*, or fore fist, is the two first knuckles of the hand, the index and middle finger knuckles. They do not share the weight of the strike evenly. The index finger takes seventy percent of the strike while the middle finger takes the remaining thirty percent.

Final rotation of the fist lifts the little finger slightly above the level plane. This emphasizes the rotation, insuring that the first two knuckles make primary contact. It is a tendency of a practitioner to put so much emphasis into the first knuckle that focusing the mind there commonly results in the little finger knuckle, as well as the other knuckles, to be positioned well below the level plane.

I once met a young martial artist who, with all the conviction in the world, explained to me how students in his school struck a metal pole to create "micro fractures" in their knuckles to make the bones stronger. A most misguided idea, certainly. An instructor who would teach this to his students is the equivalent of a flim-flam man, irresponsible, stealing from his students their time, money, and health.

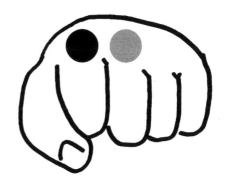

CONTACT OF STRIKING FIST: THE FIRST TWO KNUCKLES, SEVENTY AND THIRTY PERCENT.

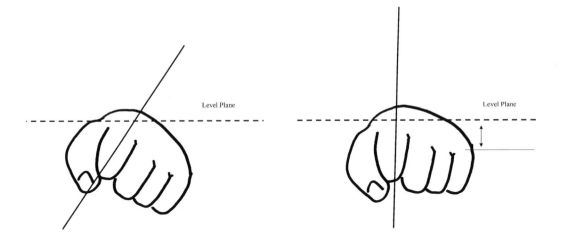

POSITION OF FIST JUST PRIOR TO CONTACT (*SEIKEN* FIST).

POSITION OF FIST UPON CONTACT, KNUCKLES NOT LEVEL (FIST PLANE – *CHINEN*).

Treat your hands and your fists with care, and act responsibly when it comes to training.

Knuckles: Test It

An easy test to establish the preferred knuckle alignment in a *seiken*, or karate fore fist, strike is to make a fist with your right hand and smack your fist into the open palm of your other hand. With a few adjustments, you should be able to smack your fist and feel the knuckles of the first two fingers take on a good hit. At this point, it is not important to have your arm and shoulder aligned because your focus is just on getting good contact with your knuckles. Do not move your slapping hand to find the correct alignment. Instead, move your fist to find the right angle for optimum contact.

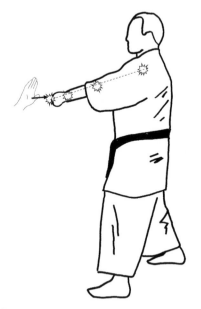

PARTNER SLAPPING FIST TO TEST PROPER ALIGNMENT.

CHAPTER SIXTEEN

The Striking Arm

Intuition and action must spring forth at the same time.

—*Taisen Deshimaru* [44]

In an overarching sense, the entire body must function together at the beginning of a strike, the middle of the process, and at the moment of impact. Because of the multiple types of joints, such as ball and hinge that are involved in the shoulder, elbow, and hand, it is important to have a firm understanding of the mechanical elements that make up these parts of the body. The understanding of the specific roles of these bones, joints, tendons, muscles, and nerves in the successful transferring of energy from your body into the opponent's body is primary. Without this understanding, the ability to generate power is greatly decreased.

1. Minimizing Shoulder Lift

When pulling the arm back into chamber in preparation for punching (*chudan tsuki*), a person should keep the following in mind.

Never lift the shoulder under the chambered fist. This is true in all forms, not just *sanchin kata*. The arm should move back into chamber with little bending of the elbow. Pulling with the bicep is incorrect because it decreases the angle between the forearm and the bicep, and usually lifts the shoulder. Moving the shoulder is an immediate tip to an opponent that you are moving.

Striking Arm: Test It 1

A drill to explore this is to take a partner and without sharing with them your intentions, face each other. Ask them to strike you in the chest from chamber, a "loaded punch" in traditional karate. It is rare that you will find a person who does not twitch their shoulder backward in an effort to gain momentum. When they twitch backward, reach out, and touch them in the chest. Simply put, when you see them prepare to punch by pulling their shoulder backward, you take advantage of it by moving, closing in on your opponent.

The second aspect of this drill it to reveal what it is you are doing and looking for, and switch places with you now as the attacker. This time, however, let your arm hang loosely at your waist and ask your partner to touch your chest the moment they see your shoulder move. You will soon see that even the slightest twitch is enough to trigger a response.

So the tactic of never lifting your shoulder can be proven empirically to be a path to more speed on your part and a two-fold increase in speed. This increase in speed comes from the better use of your own architecture by creating a faster action and because you have learned to detect intention in your attacker. You are faster because you give no indication, or forewarning of your intentions and they likely do give away their intentions.

2. Compression

Compression of the arm is important to gaining an explosive strike. By pulling the elbow back and reducing the distance between the forearm and bicep, one gives away their intentions because the shoulder is inclined to lift. By keeping the angle between the forearm and the bicep as close as possible to the original angle from the chest block, the humerus, the upper arm bone, rotates in the shoulder socket without lifting the shoulder.

Once the fist on that arm reaches its chamber, it creates a sense of compression. Pulling the arm and fist back to chamber with power slows down motion and is not necessary.

Pulling back with power also activates the shoulder area, in this instance, the group of muscles including the deltoid and trapezius, lifting the shoulder blade, the scapula, on the back.

There are many chambers for the karate fist. The most desirable chamber for *sanchin kata* is the placement of the fist at the ninth and tenth ribs and rests in front of the first floating rib. Placing the fist higher lifts the shoulder. To compensate for this high placement of the fist and to keep the shoulder low, the elbow is dropped low. This position, which is not recommended, keeps the humerus in a vertical position and places the forearm in a weak incline descending position. Neither of these solutions is superior to keeping the fist in the floating rib position.

Striking Arm: Test It 2

Place your fist high in chamber, ready to punch, directly under the pectoral muscle.

Once the fist has reached the compression stage, it then fires. This requires two things that first appear to be opposites, practice, and no thought. The practice is the first stage, tuning the movement just in the way a guitarist tunes their instrument prior to playing. The second stage is where, because the body has integrated the movement, you let the body control the action. Continuing the analogy, allowing the

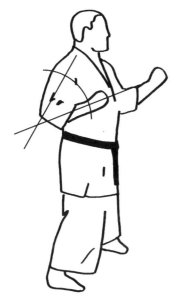

SIDE VIEW OF ACUTE ANGLE OF ELBOW, SHOULDER, AND FIST.

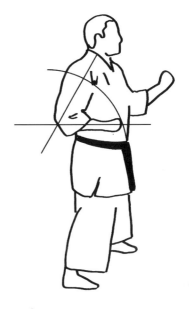

SIDE VIEW OF CORRECT ANGLE OF ELBOW, SHOULDER, AND FIST.

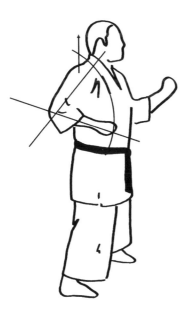

SIDE VIEW OF ACUTE ANGLE OF ELBOW, SHOULDER, AND FIST, CHAMBER TOO HIGH.

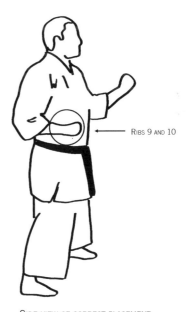

RIBS 9 AND 10

SIDE VIEW OF CORRECT PLACEMENT OF FIST ON RIBS 9 AND 10.

body to control the action is like the guitarist who never has to look at their instrument while playing because they have become so familiar with the song.

3. Staying Relaxed

Staying relaxed allows for quickness. During the first three quarters of the distance the punch covers, it is relaxed. Once the fist has passed the other fist, the rotation then begins. This exchange of fists takes place in the last quarter or so of extension toward the target.

The twisting of the fist at the last moment is important because it creates a snapping shock instead of a push punch. The twisting of the punch at the last third or so of the length the punch travels is in line with the Fibonacci Ratio in the form of a spiral. Again, this is a case of a movement that conforms to, and uses, nature instead of trying to force the body to comply with the will of the individual.

4. The Striking Fist: The Path

The striking fist goes to your centerline. This allows you to generate power via your body mass as well as to tighten the pectoral muscle, giving support to the shoulder as discussed earlier. Just as you do not want the elbow bent at contact, because it becomes a shock absorber, you do not want the shoulder to move. Allowing the twisting of the body and absorbing the power in the opposite direction of the strike is an ineffective way to transfer energy.

Striking

The fist needs to stay relaxed. Some practitioners will have a tight fist through the entirety of the punching motion, which, however, conspires to make the arm tight and thus slow. Oftentimes, the beginner will hold their fist too loosely through lack of focus or too tightly in the belief that a tight fist hits harder. The fact is the fist is held firmly, but relaxed through the punching motion and is clenched just upon contact. Compare a tight fist to a firm fist. The only detectable difference would be the yellowing of the flesh from squeezing the blood from the hand of the tight fist because the hand is held in the same position in either case.

This last-minute clenching is what Jack Dempsey,[45] former boxing champion calls, "Grabbing Tension."[46] An act similar to that of a sneeze, it makes the body like one solid piece of wood instead of a poorly constructed rickety shack. As discussed earlier, the point of contact for the fist is the first two knuckles, the index and middle finger. Primary contact, however, is made with the first, or index, knuckle.

Another way to envision this is as if you have a fresh pea in your fist. The pea is held loosely, yet secure, in the palm. When contact is made, the pea is crushed in the palm of your fist.

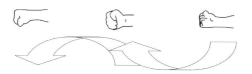

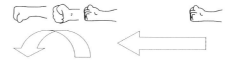

SIDE VIEW OF SPIRAL OF FIST AT CONSTANT RATE OF SPIRAL.

SIDE VIEW OF SPIRAL IN LAST SECTION OF FIBONACCI RATIO (STRETCHED SPIRAL).

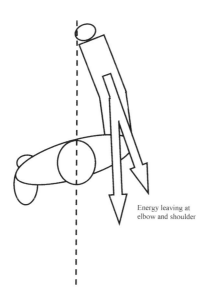

Energy leaving at elbow and shoulder

TOP VIEW SHOWING BODY ROTATION UPON IMPACT FROM NINETY-DEGREE ARM PLACEMENT.

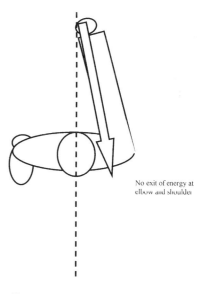

No exit of energy at elbow and shoulder

TOP VIEW SHOWING NO BODY ROTATION FROM CENTERLINE PLACEMENT OF FIST.

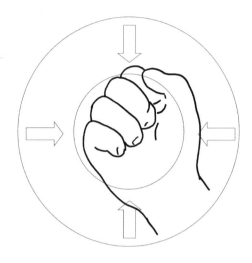

FIST CLENCHED TOO TIGHTLY.

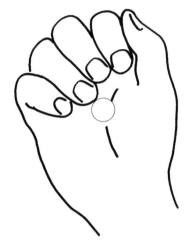

FIST HELD LOOSELY, SHOWING PEA IN HAND.

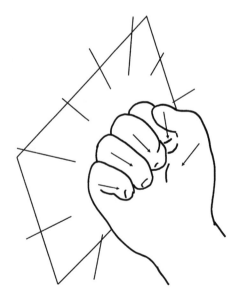

FIST CLENCHED ON CONTACT.

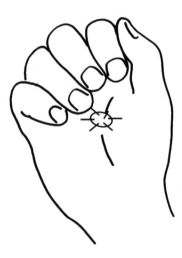

OPEN HAND SHOWING CRUSHED PEA.

When punching, the mind is placed not in the knuckles but in the wrist at the median nerve. The median nerve runs on the underside of the wrist, passing through the wrist and dividing into to several smaller nerve pathways to service the fingers. Thinking of the strike as originating from this nerve shortens your arm in your mind, giving your strike deeper penetration mechanically. It also keeps you from having to split a neurological impulse further. Your mind and energy need only go to the median nerve instead of spending effort going to the fingers that do not need to play the guitar at this moment.

The block of the *sanchin kata* is built around correct angles

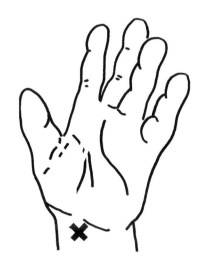

MEDIAN NERVE ON WRIST.

Striking: Test It 1

The ultimate goal of striking your opponent is the end of any further confrontation. To that end, hitting harder and faster is a serious affair and the transference of energy from your body to their body is fundamental. To test this method, you can use a large phone book or a speed pad. As air shields are designed to diffuse the power of a blow, they are not useful for this drill. Humans do not have four inches of foam surrounding their bodies.

With you and your partner facing each other in the *sanchin dachi* stance, have your partner hold the phone book on their chest. The key to transferring energy from your body to theirs is clearly the integration of the body. In this drill, however, we are going to work on the shoulder. The shoulder is among the most common places energy leaves your body and fails to transfer to their body. Strike the telephone book and at the time of impact tighten the pectoral and latissimus muscles, keeping your deltoid muscle as disengaged as possible. The deltoid muscle should have the consistency of ripe fruit, soft but not limp. Have your partner watch your shoulder. Any backward movement indicates a loss of energy and is unsatisfactory. Repeat this drill until there is no movement in the shoulder.

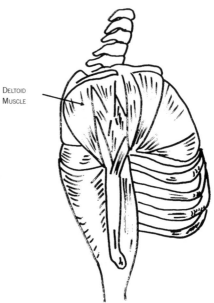

DELTOID MUSCLE

DELTOID MUSCLE (INDICATED BY ARROW).

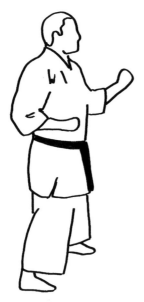

STANDING IN *SANCHIN DACHI* WITH HAND IN CHAMBER IN PREPARATION FOR STRIKE.

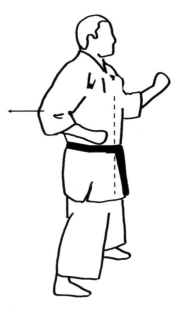

STANDING IN *SANCHIN DACHI* PULLING HAND BACKWARD IN PREPARATION FOR STRIKE.

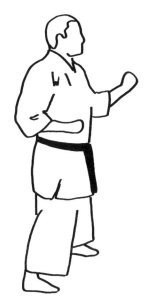

STANDING IN *SANCHIN DACHI* WITH HAND IN
CHAMBER IN PREPARATION FOR STRIKE.

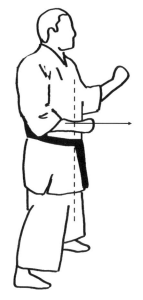

STRIKE WITH NO PREPARATION PULL.

Striking: Test It 2

Once you have achieved full transfer
of energy in the arm, that is to say, no
movement in the shoulder of the striking
arm, have your partner begin to lean into
the strike just before it arrives. This test
takes more skill and, once again, is a coop-
erative drill.

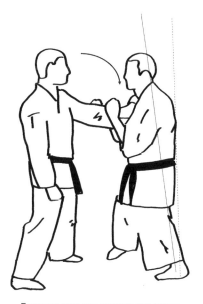

PARTNERS WITH ONE STRIKING AND OTHER
LEANING IN SLIGHTLY TO STRIKE.

CHAPTER SEVENTEEN

The Back

Go back a little to leap further.

—John Clarke [47]

The back should be held with the shoulders brought slightly forward and anchored squarely, and in a relaxed downward position. The scapula (shoulder blades) should be rolled forward and not overly so. Rolling the shoulders forward should not cave the chest because this creates a hump in the back between the shoulder blades. The action of caving the chest tampers with the structure of the spine that we are trying to achieve—a straight spine as well as the architecture of the arm as previously described. The slight rolling forward of the shoulder should create a slightly curved, but not hunched, back on the horizontal plane.

Bones, Sinew, and Muscle

The body can be broken into two structures when we talk about striking, or making contact with an opponent. Those two structures can be considered the bow and the string of a bow used for shooting arrows. The bow is equal to the bones and the string is equal to the tendons or sinew. The bow can only be used in the capacity of a weapon as a club without its string. Just as a bow is useless without the string, the bone is the same without the sinew. In addition, like a bow the bones are powerful when put into the proper architecture. Architecture implies relationship and the power lays in the relationship of bone to bone first, secondly the relationship of sinew to sinew, and, finally, the concerted effort of the sinew and the organized architecture of the bones. When erecting a tent, the first thing that is done is the poles are put into place, or in the bones. Afterward, the stakes are used to make the tent taut via ropes, again in the body the sinew. This elegant structure can now withstand wind, rain, and other elements that may assault it. These two examples demonstrate the need for proper alignment. The sinew, in this example the tent ropes, is worthless without the bow and the tent is a mess without the poles. They must work together for success.

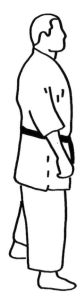

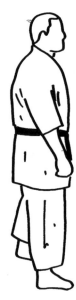

SIDE VIEW OF TORSO STANDING NATURALLY.

SIDE VIEW OF TORSO STANDING WITH SLIGHT
HUNCH OF *SANCHIN KATA* STANCE.

This principle is applicable to both small, such as a pup tent, or larger platforms, such as the Seven Wonders of the World. The Seven Wonders of the Ancient World are usually agreed as: the Hanging Gardens of Babylon, the Statue of Zeus at Olympia, the Temple of Artemis at Ephesus, the Mausoleum at Halicarnassus, The Colossus of Rhodes, the Pharos (Lighthouse) of Alexandria, and the Pyramids of Egypt.

The Colossus of Rhodes, a statue in the shape of a man, was said to be so large that it ships sailed between its legs as they entered the harbor. The Pharos (Lighthouse) of Alexandria was a beacon seen for miles and miles at sea. The other wonders were all great works in their own ways as well, yet only one exists today. The Pyramids of Egypt were once covered with marble and a cap made of gold, and said to be blinding in the Egyptian sun. Yet even without the cosmetics of the marble and the gold, the structure still stands because it is naturally stable. The analogy is clear: *sanchin kata* should be and is the same in that it is not based on gilding or affectation but in tried and true practicality, structural integrity, and knowledgeable application.

For those who choose to pursue *sanchin kata*, fundamental stability is essential.

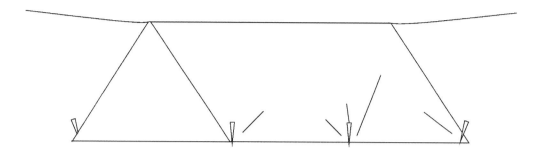

PUP TENT.

Chapter Eighteen

The Energetic and Mechanical Structure

Any sufficiently advanced technology is indistinguishable from magic.

—*Arthur C. Clarke* [48]

The perception of *ki* can be many things because it varies with the level of skill the practitioner possesses—think of it as quality and quantity. The scientific method asks that we take a subject, break it down to its smallest element, test it, record the results, and then repeat it again. This is science, definable, and repeatable. When you can define and repeat an experiment, an item, the subject of the experiment then becomes quantitative and qualitative, it is defined.

The quality and quantity of *ki* is difficult to define. *Ki* has a quality that cannot be tested in a true scientific method and since it cannot be tested in a scientific method, to the scientific mind it does not exist.

Ki has a quantity but it cannot be put into a jar. This leaves the nature of *ki* to be one of experience, and making it more difficult to define a personal one as well. A personal experience is difficult to relate and is based on assumptions.

An example of assuming a personal experience is strawberries. Frankly, I do not care for them, yet many people love strawberries and they are perplexed when I say I do not care for them. They assume the taste that they experience is the same one I have, but it is not. Nobody knows what any food tastes like to another person. We can only assume a commonality of experience. The same is true of *ki*. The quality of the strawberries taste and the quality of *ki* are difficult to truly know.

Sometimes we are asked to make a leap in our thinking process, a leap that propels us in the direction of a target we presume to be authentic. Science will tell you for something to be real; it must be definable, observable, and repeatable. The Big Bang, the assumed origin of the universe is not definable, not observable, and clearly not repeatable, yet it is printed in textbooks and discussed as fact.

Therefore, the leap to accepting the existence of *ki* is a personal one, as amorphous as the Big Bang, and as personal as a strawberry—all complicated by the skill, the individual, the environment, and assumptions.

Simply put, *ki* energy is not a panacea, not a trump card, and not the holy grail of all forms of martial arts. *Ki* is part of the package. It is important in that it helps sustain and aid the practitioner, but if it is the sole means by which you choose to define your martial arts, then you will be disappointed and possibly hurt quite badly. In the three levels of a confrontation, escape, control, and martial, *ki* is never the primary means of execution.

Ki, which refers to the body's vital energy, is generally defined as "life force" or "spiritual energy". This vital energy, recognized in numerous cultures, is called by many names: *qi* in Chinese, *ki* in Japanese, *prana* when spoken of by a Hindu, and *pneuma* in Greek. To understand fully the practice of *sanchin kata*, it is essential to touch upon this energy, which is widely accepted to be an integral part of the *kata* as well as of many forms of martial arts. Certainly, there are those in the martial arts community who do not recognize the existence of *ki*. We will discuss how that energy is considered by many to manifest itself, and its purpose and value to the martial arts and *sanchin kata*.

Ki energy is not a magic trick used to stop an attacker. Rather, it allows, among other things, a practitioner to harness additional energy for increased power in execution and to withstand blows. The stories that follow, while really a series of what one would call "parlor tricks," provide excellent examples of how *ki* energy can be used.

In the early eighties, I was a student at a Pac 10 School on the West Coast. The school at that time was nationally ranked in track and field, and had one of the greatest cross-country runners in the world. I found myself taking a physical education class from one of the track coaches. One class, about midway through the quarter, while talking about athletic performance, he began to tell an odd story about another coach whom he worked with who used a form of energetic manipulation to win bar bets. The instructor went on to explain that while on trips to track meets both in the United States and abroad, the other coach would seek out bets at bars where the coaches would congregate. The bet was simple; he could beat you at arm wrestling. Once the bet was made, he then prepared the opponent. This preparation involved disrupting the opponents *ki* there were several methods the coach employed. One was to wave his hand back and forth in a horizontal motion over the opponent's solar plexus, after which the coach would arm-wrestle and win, often against a larger opponent.

Our physical education teacher and track coach then set out to show a classroom of college students how to go about replicating the disruption of another person's *ki* energy. Within moments, the classroom was paired off and we were manipulating each other's *ki*, making each other go weak, testing it, resorting the energy, and then testing again.

The Test It below demonstrates the way we were shown to diminish and restore another person's energy. There are many other ways to do this test, some more impressively than this demonstration. However, in keeping with example, the information is presented without any additions or deletions in technique.

Energetic Structure: Test It

This is a two-person drill in which a tester and a subject are needed. The subject begins by simply standing still at rest with their arms at their sides, in a casual manner. The subject then holds either arm out from their body, to the side, at ninety degrees. The tester then reaches up and tries to push the arm back down to the subject's side. This is not a battle and the push needs to only be a second or two, just to establish strength and not actually power the arm back into place, although sometimes that can happen. Have the subject return to the resting position, and then with your right hand wave your fingertips back and forth across the sternum of the subject in a "Z" pattern about three times swiftly.

Have the subject place their arm in the same ninety-degree position they previously used and again try to move their arm downward to their side. It should be weakened and move with ease.

Option: Instead of waving your hand in a "Z" pattern, blow a stream of cigarette smoke into the same area. All other parts of the test remain the same.

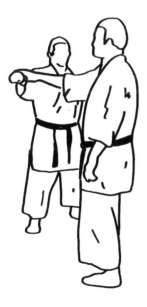

STANDING WITH RIGHT ARM OUT IN
PREPARATION FOR PUSHING DOWN.

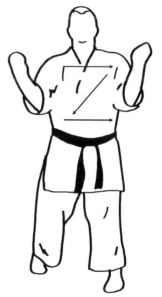

STANDING NATURALLY WITH PARTNER
MAKING "Z" ACROSS CHEST.

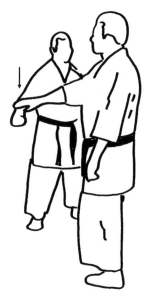

ARM PUSHED DOWN.

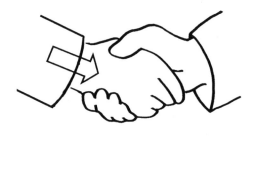

HANDSHAKE GRIP TO RESTORE WITH PULL.

Once having tested the subject in the weakened state, you can restore their energy several ways. One method is the handshake. Take their right hand as if shaking hands, and then grab their arm just above their wrist holding their arm still with your left hand gently pull their hand toward yourself as if trying to separate the hand from the arm at the wrist. Next, wiggle the hand up and down five or six times. Repeat the process on the other side. Once you have done both hands, test the subject's arm again. You will find that his strength has returned.

In another arm-testing situation similar to that described in the account of the track coach took place. This event involved a powerfully built *kung fu* practitioner who was also in the United States

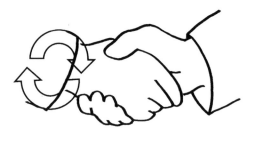

HANDSHAKE GRIP TO RESTORE WITH VERTICAL MOTION.

Army. In a room of some thirty-odd martial artists ranging in age, skill, and style, the presenter, also a *kung fu* practitioner asked the Army member to stand and put his arm into the air at the ninety-degree angle like the track coach had done to the college students. The presenter tested the Army member's arm for strength in the same way, but then the event took a different turn. The practitioner stepped across the room turned, pointed his hand, and gave a shout. He walked back and asked the Army member to put his arm back in the air and with little effort, and two fingers, pushed the arm to the Army member's side. After some brief discussion and a demonstration on reversing the energy, a person from the audience asked the Army guy what had happened, his reply was, "I couldn't keep my arm up, and I am kind of half pissed about it."

So can people fail miserably when applying *ki*? Yes? Can they succeed? Yes, albeit under controlled situations with a compliant partner. A member of a Corrections Emergency Response Team, one of the officers who break up jail fights, told me in so many words to always default to the mechanical. What he means is a pressure point may not work for many reasons. Some reasons for failure of pressure points are: the attacker being on drugs, not being able to find the pressure point, and some other reasons you can probably list yourself.

Pain compliance is creating enough pain to make an attacker dance on their toes while you lead them to the door. It is important to understand that pain compliance may not work because the attacker may not feel the pain the way others do. However, immobilization is the mechanical means of actually locking a joint or pinning a person to the point of total control; now that is very difficult to fight.

Mechanical Structure: Test It 1

Have a partner lie face down on the ground and hold their arms out to the side as if flying. Place your left palm on their right elbow. Have them place their left hand palm up. Grip the back of their left hand, so the palm of your left hand is on the knuckles of their left hand, and then bend their wrist making the fingers point skyward. Now, place your right hand on their forearm, pressing down and pinning their arm to the floor. Once you have set this position, have them attempt to escape.

Mechanical Structure: Test It 2

Have a partner lie face down on the ground again and hold their arms out to the side as if flying. Place your left knee on their right elbow. Have them place their right hand palm up. Grip the back of their right hand, so your palm is on the knuckles of their backhand and bend the wrist, making the fingers point skyward. Once you have set this position, have them attempt to escape.

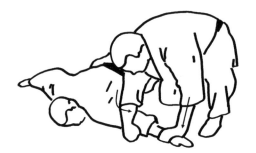

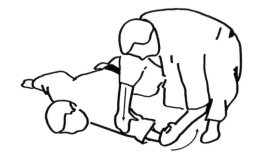

ARM-TO-ARM PIN OF PARTNER TO THE GROUND AS IF FLYING.

INSET OF HAND-TO-HAND SHOWING
FINGERS POINTED SKYWARD.

Mechanical Structure: Test It 3

Have a partner lie face down on the ground again and hold their arms out to the side as if flying. Place your feet on each side of the left elbow while squatting like a baseball catcher over their left arm facing their left hand. With both of your hands, scoop under your partner's arm at the wrist, one of your hands covering the other. Finally, sit on their triceps, the muscles between their shoulder and elbow. The motions are to sit and lift. Do this slowly and with caution. Have them once again attempt an escape.

The results of these three attempts, Version One—extremity-to-extremity pin, Version Two—inner extremity (knee)-to-extremity and Version Three—core-to-extremity, move from negligible control to

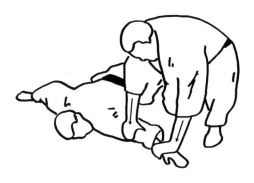

HAND-TO-ARM PIN OF PARTNER TO THE GROUND AS IF FLY-ING.

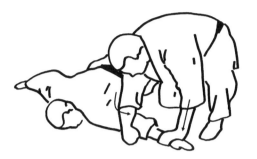

ARM-TO-ARM PIN OF PARTNER TO THE GROUND AS IF FLYING.

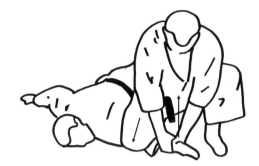

KNEE ON BACK OF ELBOW.

definitive control. If your opponent is able to move their core, the center of their body, they have an opportunity to escape the hold. In the same way that you are controlling their core, you must have a strong core, a *sanchin kata*-strong core whether you are standing, as preferred in karate, or on the ground submitting to a pin for test purposes. Having a strong core and executing movement from that strong core are the very essence of *sanchin kata* and ultimately karate.

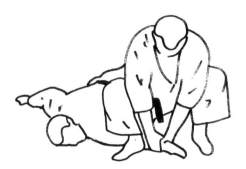

SQUATTING OVER THE PARTNER'S ELBOW.

CHAPTER NINETEEN

The Iron Shirt

*Ability is what you're capable of doing. Motivation determines
what you do. Attitude determines how well you do it.*

—*Lou Holtz* [49]

Envisioning *ki* energy surrounding particular parts of the body can be very helpful in *sanchin kata* to concentrate power and create a protection of the internal
organs. Pressure needs to exert from the abdomen at all times during the *kata*. Rather
than focusing just on the belly, the front, one needs to be mindful of exerting pressure on all sides, the left, right, and rear. Approximately one hand width below the
belly button is the location of the *hara*, the Japanese term for what is considered the
location of an individual's being. Mentally circling the waist at this level, one then
expands with the breath the belly, the sides of the abdomen, and the kidney area.
Once expanded, it is then set in place with a dropping of the barrel to anchor or fix-
ate the lower abdomen. At this point, the abdomen should physically have dropped
as well.

For the entire torso, an "Iron Shirt" can be envisioned. This Iron Shirt is also
locked down and fixed in place, and the entire area covered by the Iron Shirt in a
state of expansive tension. Once the lower abdomen has been set, that is to say, the
barrel has been dropped, the breath is lowered, and the skeletal architecture put into
place. Take a deep breath in and expand the lower abdomen, the *hara*, and hold that
position. Once expanded, the lower abdomen does not retract. Now while breathing,
it may look like the abdomen is moving in and out but the lower abdomen, around
the belt knot, does not move. Hold the lower abdomen, the *hara*, as if it is where an
inflated tire that this expanded pressure does not change. This expansive tension
keeps the focus on the lower part of the body and keeps it strong. The sensation one
should attempt to achieve is that of an industrial tire filled to its proper level of air.
Just as a modern truck tire is composed of bands of steel cables, treated rubber, fiber-
glass, and other products, the body has a complex layering of materials that offer a
combination of strength, flexibility, and protection. As you move through the body
from front to back at the ribs, you move through the epidermis, the outer layer of

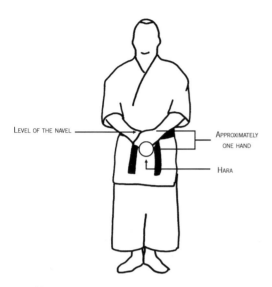

LEVEL OF THE NAVEL

APPROXIMATELY
ONE HAND

HARA

HAND HELD AGAINST BODY AT NAVEL INDICATING THE *HARA*.

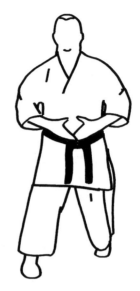

HAND HELD WIDE TO INDICATE WIDTH AND WRAP OF
NATURAL BELLY PRIOR TO EXPANSION OF ABDOMEN.

skin, the dermis, the layer that contains the sweat glands and the hypodermis, holding fat and blood vessels. As you transfer to the muscles and bone, you find thicker and stronger elements. A tire inflated and run within its boundaries will perform without concern by the driver for some fifty thousand miles. The tire will absorb and rebound from bumps, rocks, and curbs. Your outer body is also constructed with similar intent; it is your responsibility to inflate and operate the body correctly.

The Iron Shirt is based, in part, on intent. The intent is not to allow a strike to penetrate the body. There is an architectural, mental, and spiritual aspect.

The architectural aspect of the Iron Shirt has been established earlier. The architecture is critical, ranging from the feet up through the legs and radiating throughout the body. Once the architecture is in place, the intent takes place. Simply saying, "I will block the strike from entering my body" does not work by itself. The Iron Shirt provides the necessary architecture on which to launch the intent Iron Shirt. Mechanically, the abdomen must be crunched together in a manner similar to the stacking of poker chips. Imagine taking a stack of poker chips in your hand and hold the stack over the table, maybe only a poker chip's width from the tabletop. Now drop each chip rapidly, one by one, on top of one another. Click, click, and click they go in order, falling a short distance, and quickly coming to rest on the one below. This is the way the torso needs to order itself. To be structurally sound for *sanchin*

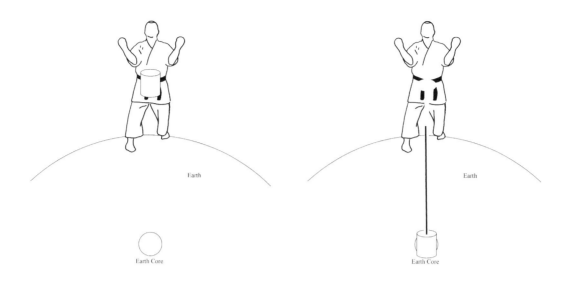

IMAGE OF BARREL IN ABDOMEN.

IMAGE OF BARREL DROPPING THROUGH
BODY AND ANCHORING TO CORE OF EARTH.

kata, the torso must fall into place in a specific order. If one were to grab stack of poker chips between thumb and forefinger, and then pinch, uneven pressure would be created. Eventually, with enough pressure, the middle chips would shoot out the backside of the stack. Again, the stack of chips is analogous to your torso and crunching down the front of your body is equivalent to the pinching of the poker chip stack. By creating an unequal pressure on the front side of the spine and making the practitioner hunch unduly, thereby making the practitioner imbalanced and weak.

Using the four points of the compass, one can "spark off" intent outward away from the body. The sensation in the body begins at the waist level, around the belt, or *obi*. Some people simply envision arrows such as those seen on a mechanical drawing, others may employ such visualizations as a shield, or an energy burst—the choice is up to the individual.

The method is as follows: Standing in *sanchin dachi*, use the four points of the compass and slowly create the sensation of expansion in the lower abdomen, not just in front but outward from all sides of the body. Eventually all four points will become one motion. As you begin, however, start with the abdomen and once set, move to the sides of the body simultaneously, East and West. Finally, move to the back, at the lower spine and expand outward there as well. Once that sensation is in place, extend it upward to the chest, under the armpits and to the spine area between

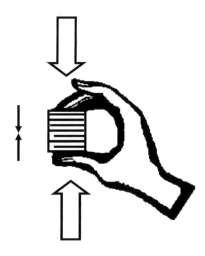

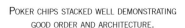

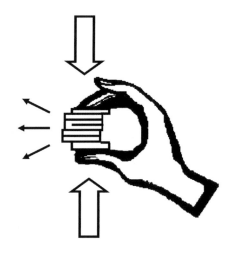

POKER CHIPS STACKED WELL DEMONSTRATING
GOOD ORDER AND ARCHITECTURE.

POKER CHIPS STACKED POORLY AND
SHOWING FRAGILE ARCHITECTURE.

the shoulder blades.

The Iron Shirt, once set, creates balance and unity within the body, allowing the practitioner to explode with exceptional power in the direction of the strike.

Iron Shirt, The Beginning: Test It 1

Stand in *sanchin dachi* and *morote chudan kumae,* and have a partner face you. Your partner is going to drop a punch into the top of your chest. The goal is to test the stance, not how hard your partner can strike. Note to the striker: The punch for these purposes needs to be done in this fashion: the striking part of the fist needs to employ the entire surface of the fist, using all knuckles. This is not a normal karate strike. The strike needs to be dead; that is, when it makes contact, the inertia

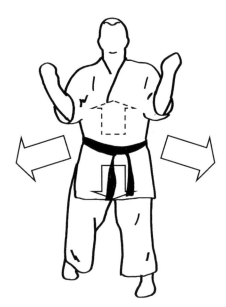

DIRECTIONS OF ENERGY INTENT.

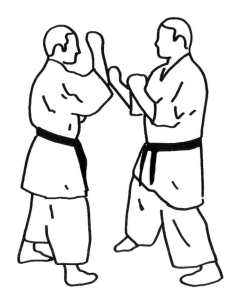
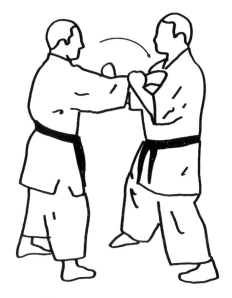

TWO PARTNERS FACING EACH OTHER, ONE IN *SANCHIN KATA* AND THE OTHER WITH HAMMER FIST READY TO STRIKE.

HAMMER FIST DROPPED INTO THE CHEST MUSCLE (PECTORAL) OF THE RECEIVING PARTNER.

of the strike is the only penetration. There is no pushing involved. To help achieve this, once the fist makes contact with the upper pectoral muscle, leave it in contact with the other person for a brief moment. A person could liken it to having a wet, balled-up towel thrown at their chest by a baseball pitcher.

For the person being tested, assemble your architecture, preparing for the strike. Upon contact, you will need to have your Iron Shirt in place. At the moment of contact, expel energy outward toward the strike. Note that the entire body needs to be unified. Simply leaning into the strike will impede the transfer of power. Any twisting, dropping, or leaning will only weaken the *sanchin dachi* stance. When I was first learning this technique, my instructor would hold his hands to his head and sweep them down his body while saying in his Japanese accent, "Wood, whole body, one piece of wood." This is the mental imagery needed for this test and drill.

The sensations are your keys to correct application. For the person striking, they should feel a rejection of their strike. The person being tested should feel no penetration. The strike should hit the surface and not enter the body. Note to the striker: The sensations that you feel are very important to the person being tested. Give input as to the depth, twist, power, or any significant sensation you may feel on your end of the experience, both positive and negative. This feedback is very helpful in learning to generate an effective Iron Shirt quickly.

Because the striker is using a flat, dead strike, it is possible to do this drill for the duration of a normal class without injury.

Iron Shirt, Intermediate: Test It 2

Standing in *sanchin dachi*, drop your hands to your side and establish the Iron Shirt. As the striker makes contact with your chest, lift a hand and quickly tap them on their chest. The goal of this drill is to keep the Iron Shirt intact and yet be flexible enough to smoothly and quickly strike back. Over time, modify your movement to touch them with your fingertips prior to their hand making light contact with you. Light but firm contact is required for this drill.

Note: The open-hand fingertips used to tap the opponent's chest in this drill helps teach speed first and avoid any incidental heavy contact with a fist. However, a fist may be used for this drill by people with higher skill levels and more control.

Iron Shirt, Advanced: Test It 3

Standing in *sanchin dachi*, hold your hands downward to the side and allow your partner to strike your abdomen. Again, this is about architecture, not about how tight you can clench your abdomen muscles. If the Iron Shirt is in place, you should experience little or no discomfort.

Iron Shirt, Advanced: Test It 4

Standing in *sanchin dachi,* hold your hands upward into the position of two

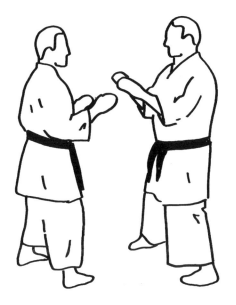

TWO PARTNERS FACING EACH OTHER.

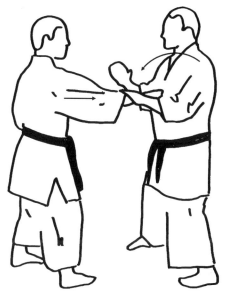

AS ONE PARTNER STRIKES, THE OTHER ATTEMPTS TO TOUCH THE ATTACKER'S CHEST AS SWIFTLY AS POSSIBLE.

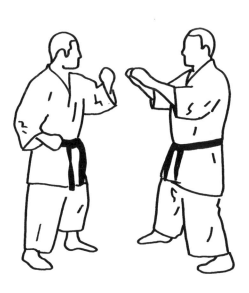

TWO PARTNERS FACING EACH OTHER.

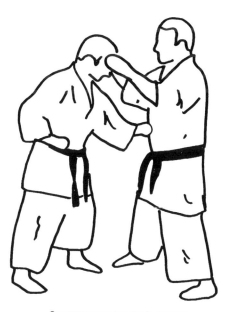

ONE STRIKING THE OTHER'S ABDOMEN WITH ROUNDHOUSE PUNCHES.

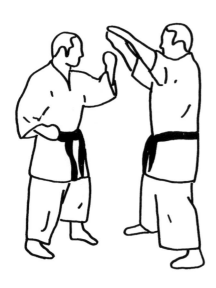

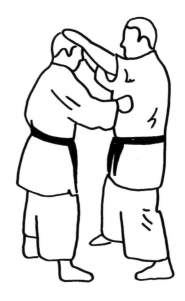

TWO PARTNERS FACING EACH OTHER AND ONE WITH ARMS
HELD UPWARD AT SHOULDER HEIGHT OR HIGHER.

ARMS HELD HIGH WITH PARTNER STRIKING TORSO.

open-hand head blocks and allow your partner to strike your abdomen. Again, this
is about architecture. Be forewarned that in this instance, you are lifting your arms
and in doing so, the nature of the body is to un-stack itself. The body has a tendency to open up. It takes discipline to keep the *sanchin dachi* architecture and Iron Shirt
in place. This form of practice is recommended only for those confident in their abilities.

Chapter Twenty

Rooting

There is nothing so easy to learn as experience and nothing so hard to apply.

—*Josh Billings* [50]

When executing *sanchin kata*, the concept of rooting or anchoring oneself to the ground is essential to maintaining powerful stances and remaining in balance throughout. This action, however, is invisible to the eye. It is about setting the Iron Shirt and the body's architecture in place, and envisioning that energy extending into the ground, in essence, creating energetic roots. The transparent nature of this rooting is critical, and should not be confused with "gripping" the ground, as is sometimes seen. By gripping, rather than rooting to the ground, a person can be easily displaced because there is no depth involved. By the same token, any gripping motion, whether with hands or feet, is not desired because it serves as a giveaway to one's intentions.

My judo instructor Kenji Yamada, a back-to-back national champion in the fifties, would only lightly grasp my *gi* when demonstrating a technique. In fact, he often just used the last two fingers, the little and ring, on the lapel of his opponent. Yamada *Sensei* taught us that if he gripped hard his opponent would know his intentions. Using a light grasp, one trades power for superior technique. When performing *sanchin kata*, this example should be considered as well.

Rooting: Test It 1

Stand in *morote sanchin kumae* (*sanchin dachi* and double chest blocks) and grip the ground with your toes, twisting your feet into the ground. The edges of your feet should be pale from the pressure and your toes the same. Often this is stage is referred to "gripping the ground," and is not quite correct in that gripping implies to grab so an attempt to grab the ground with the toes is made. In actuality, the feet seize the ground by using adhesion. Trying to grab the ground with the toes actually weakens the stance. When you are ready, have your partner give slow, steady, and consistently increasing pressure with their fist on your chest in order to displace you. Next, stand as described at the beginning of the chapter—firm, heavy and rooted, relaxing into the proper architecture of the feet, shins, knees, thighs, waist, and torso, including the four points of the spine (sacrum, lumbar, thoracic, and cervical bones). Then have your partner repeat the same test, steady and with increasing pressure.

Rooting: Test It 2

Repeat the same test, this time having your partner push sharply and quickly with intent to displace your stance.

The end result should be clear in that rooting to the ground is not based on a hard tensile strength, but heavy anchored strength based in a unified body.

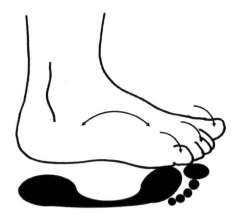

FOOT WITH TOES GRIPPING.

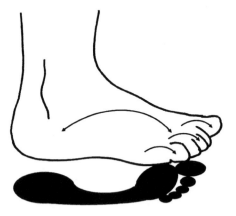

FOOT WITH TOES RELAXED GRIPPING.

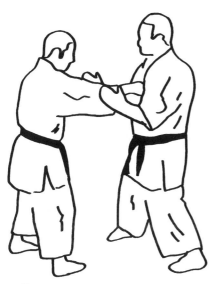

Two partners face each other in *SANCHIN DACHI* in preparation to gripping ground.

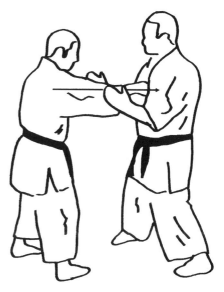

Person being tested receiving pressure from vertical fist on chest.

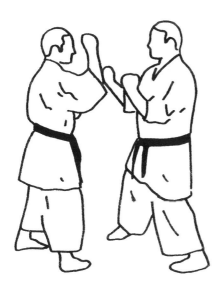

Standing in *SANCHIN KATA* with standing fist just short of the other person's chest.

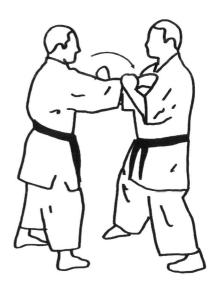

Tapping the other person's chest with standing fist.

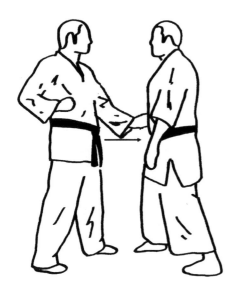

TWO PEOPLE PREPARING TO TEST STEPPING IN
SANCHIN KATA WITH FIST TO BELT KNOT.

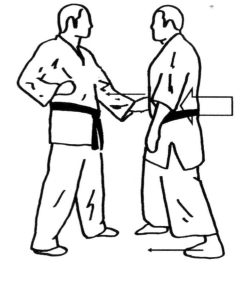

STEPPING FORWARD AND HAVING FIST AND ARM PROVIDE
HYDRAULIC PRESSURE AGAINST FORWARD MOVEMENT.

Two-Person Drill: Hydraulic Fist to the Abdomen.

Standing in *sanchin dachi,* place both hands in front of you in a chest block, a *chudan uke.* Have your partner stand in front of you and to the outside so their shoulder meets your centerline. Now, have your partner place their fist in a vertical orientation on your lower abdomen, the *koshi,* with their arm bent. The goal is to practice good technique while stepping. The partner's arm should provide pressure against the stepping motion, and only enough to test the structure of your movement. If you are being stopped completely from moving then your partner needs to give less pressure and build up to more over time. The partner's fist needs to act as a lever, not an anchor.

CHAPTER TWENTY-ONE

The Mind

Your mind is what makes everything else work.

—*Kareem Abdul-Jabbar* [51]

Philosophers and psychologists have argued about the nature of the human mind for centuries. One version of the definition or concept of the mind is the substantial view. The substantial view makes the argument that the mind is its own entity, which stands apart from the brain. The idea of the mind being different from the brain was championed by Plato. This premise, the substantial view, makes the mind the seat of consciousness and the brain the interface by which the mind exerts its will.

The other view of the mind/brain or brain is the functional view. This functional view holds that the mind is really just a label used to order an assortment of mental functions that do not have a great level of commonality other than the fact that the brain is aware of them. This design was advocated by Aristotle.[52] As discussed at the outset of this book, recognition of the mind/body connection is critical to the understanding of *sanchin kata* and to the martial arts in general.

Brain Waves

There are four levels of brain activity: beta, alpha, theta, and delta. Brain waves are scientifically recorded by measuring the fluctuating electrical impulses in the brain. Beta waves range from 14 to 30 cycles per second. Such pulses are indicative of a person who is fully awake, alert, excited, or tense. Alpha waves run from 8 to 13 cycles per second. They are characterized by deep relaxation, passive awareness, or a composed state of mind. Theta waves range from 4 to 7 cycles per second. They are indicative of a person who is drowsy, unconscious, or in a state of deep tranquility. Delta waves run from 0.5 to 3.5 cycles per second. They are characterized by sleep, unawareness, or deep unconsciousness.

The first two levels, beta and alpha, are the ones we are concerned with in martial arts. The brain discharges beta waves when we are awake and intentionally focused. We are alert, ready for action, even irritated or afraid. This is because we are in an active mind state. Beta is not as useful as alpha to the martial artist because it

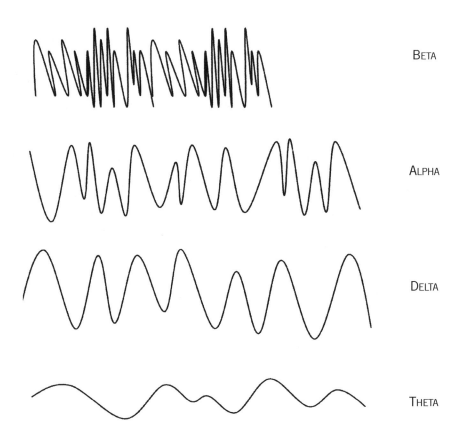

BETA

ALPHA

DELTA

THETA

CHART OF BRAIN WAVE FREQUENCIES.

is about thinking and thinking quite frequently gets you hit. The alpha state is indicative of physical and mental relaxation, the relaxed, but alert mind. It is usually achieved during meditation. In the alpha state, we are aware of what is happening around us yet ultra-focused in our concentration; this can be referred to as the creative state. The professional athlete would call it being "in the zone," or being "in the flow." We have all heard of athletes who while facing great impediments to their game such as the flu, an injury, or a tragedy have excelled beyond what was expected. A large part of their success and performance directly results from an ability to shift into an alpha state of consciousness during competition In 1984, Marcus Allen won the National Football League's Super Bowl XVIII Most Valuable Player award. In interviews after the event, he spoke about being in the zone. I paraphrase his comments, but he knew that the day was different outside of it being the National Football League's Super Bowl, he spoke of how the other players on the field seemed to move in slow motion and he had insight to what the other players where going to do next. It was truly an experience that goes beyond the words to explain it.

A guess on my part would be the reader has experienced incidences of non-lucid action yourself, spontaneous and unique. It could have been a potential car accident, the dropping of a knife while cooking, playing music, or a sporting activity. Non-lucid action is that time when you, like Marcus Allen, felt in control, yet part of something bigger and time was experienced differently.

One of the benefits to training in martial arts is the ability to switch between beta (waking brain waves) and alpha (or "the zone") brain waves. Multiple studies have shown that world-class athletes, no matter what their sport, have the ability to switch their brain waves almost instantly from beta to alpha. In martial arts, this sort of thing is demonstrated all the time. Breaking techniques are a good example. Concentration begins as the hand moves into chamber. By the time a practitioner's fist strikes the board or the brick, his or her mind is fully in an alpha state. The target shatters effortlessly.

A traditional martial arts concept, *zanshin*, involves the brain in an alpha state. Defined as "continuing mind," *zanshin* is a state of enhanced awareness that should exist just before, during, and after combat. A practitioner in this state should be hyper-aware of his or her surroundings and prepared for anything. He or she is working in an alpha state. A refined sense of *zanshin* can even help practitioners avoid conflict altogether.

The Mind: Test It

Controlling the body has often been encapsulated in the phrase, "Mind over matter." The overt point of the statement is that the mind, under proper attitude or intent, can control the body. This time we are going to use the body to control the mind. Standing in *sanchin dachi* with your hands at your sides, place your tongue on the roof of your mouth. Close your eyes and roll them to the top of your head, and hold them in that position for a couple of seconds. Note the sensation in your brain. Keeping your eyes closed, quickly return your eyes to the forward-looking position, and again note the sensation. After allowing your brain to clear, roll your eyes upward again. While holding the position, sense the brain shift. This is the alpha state, the creative state. Releasing feel yourself settle back into the beta state. You can now move at will from beta to alpha and back by using the eye roll.[53] Another example of the body controlling the mind that is more common is the athlete who gets a season-ending injury. Depression often follows because of the loss of a goal, team comradeship, or simply disappointment. If you think back to a time when you where injured and unable to participate in the training at the *dojo*, you may have well experienced your body and its injury bring on a level of depression.

An example of the positive side of this brain controlling the body is when you

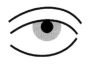

ALPHA EYE ROLLS BEGINNING IN NATURAL POSITION.   ALPHA EYE ROLLS WITH EYES ROTATED UPWARD.

receive a good word from a friend, a co-worker, or superior. These comments can change the nature of your body. You may walk faster, be happier, or even sit straighter in your chair. All of these are positive manifestations of a thought from one person, made into words, projected through the air and into your brain where the sounds are translated to words and then ideas, and they change your body in a positive way.

Chapter Twenty-Two
Ten-Minute Sanchin Kata

In the midst of movement and chaos, keep stillness inside of you.

—*Deepak Chopra, MD* [54]

The customary method of testing *sanchin kata* is called *shime*. This form of testing involves two people, one performing the *kata* and an assistant who strikes the performers body at times of contraction and exertion over the body. This form of testing is usually fast, the strikes are done quickly and with deliberation.

Ten-minute *sanchin kata* is a version of *sanchin kata* testing that is different from what is customarily taught.

This version does not involve striking the person being tested, the practitioner. It is executed slowly, focusing solely on form, rather than the power aspects of *sanchin kata*. The goal is to allow the person doing the *kata* to concentrate on achieving unification of the body and, without time constraints, be able to correct their position, and feel the proper form at each step of the way.

Excessive power or speed is not needed. Power and speed are not used in ten-minute *sanchin kata*. Practice is done with an eye toward perfection of technique and not how fast or strong the person being tested can be.

The tester does not strike the practitioner's body. There is no trickery or overt striking involved. The tester and the practitioner are acting in a symbiotic relationship to ultimately aid the practitioner in achieving a better understanding of the *kata* and their own body.

Each area on the body can be tested in eight directions as shown in the diagram of *happo no kuzushi*; however, often just the main four directions, North, East, South, and West are needed.

The test begins by having practitioner assume the *morote chudan kamae* position, or *sanchin dachi* with two chest blocks. The tester stands in front of the person in *sanchin dachi* and begins by covering the fists of the practitioner with their open hand. The tester then pulls the fists away from the practitioner, but gently enough that they just barely move. This position is held for a minute or two; the time is at the discretion of the tester. Again, it is important for the tester to keep in mind that

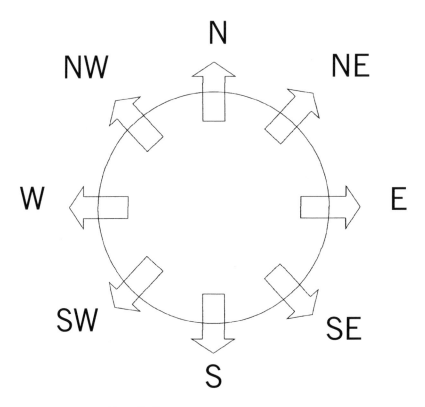

HAPPO NO KUZUSHI, THE EIGHT POINTS OF IMBALANCE.

the effort needed to just begin to break the form is all that is needed.

The reasoning behind this is once the form of the *kata* is broken, in other words, the architecture of the position, there is no point to continuing the test. If this happens, do not continue, as the lesson is lost. Simply reset with the proper corrections and proceed.

The tester then moves to the second position of the test by sliding their palms on to the knuckles of the practitioner's fist and again giving pressure to the hand pushing them into toward the body of the practitioner. This position can be held as long as needed and pressure can vary.

Next, the tester moves their hands to the outside of the practitioner's hands, the thumb side, and pressure is given inward.

Finally, the tester moves to the inside, or little-finger side and pressure is applied outward.

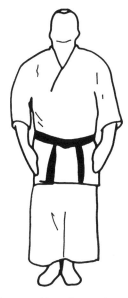

ATTENTION MOVEMENT: NONE. BREATH: IN THROUGH NOSE, RELEASE THROUGH MOUTH, SHALLOW).

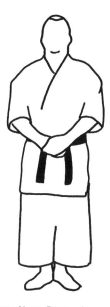

YOI (MOVEMENT: NONE. BREATH: IN THROUGH NOSE, RELEASE THROUGH MOUTH, SHALLOW).

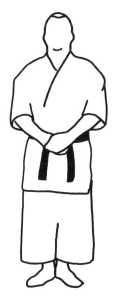

YOI (MOVEMENT: NONE. BREATH: IN THROUGH NOSE, RELEASE THROUGH MOUTH, DEEPER, HALF OF YOUR MAXIMUM CAPACITY).

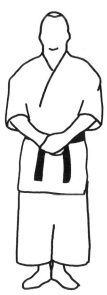

YOI, BREATHING (MOVEMENT: NONE. BREATH: IN THROUGH NOSE, RELEASE THROUGH MOUTH, DEEPER, MAXIMUM CAPACITY).

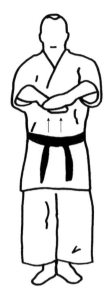

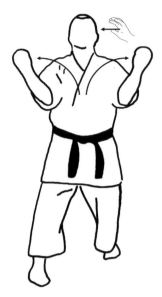

RAISING HANDS IN PREPARATION (MOVEMENT: ARMS ONLY. BREATH: IN THROUGH NOSE).

MOROTE KAMAE HEAD: RIGHT PALM TO LEFT TEMPLE (MOVEMENT: RIGHT STEP FORWARD TO SANCHIN DACHI. BREATH: IN THROUGH NOSE, RELEASE THROUGH MOUTH).

Now that the pattern, principle, and technique are understood, the other areas of testing are:

The Head: forehead, both temples and the back of the head

The Fists/Arms: push, pull, side to side.

The Torso: sternum, both shoulders (pressing into the shoulder toward the other shoulder), and the back between the shoulder blades.

The Waist: front, back, side to side.

The Thighs: outside to inside, there is no inside to outside; front of lead leg, front to back.

Calves: The calves are tested back to front and the front, or shins, are tested just below the kneecap pushing back. The calves can also be tested by leg to leg, or tester's hands to practitioners.

Feet: back, front, side to side, and twisting.

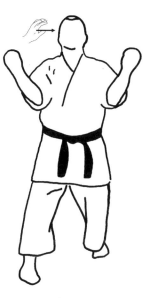

MOROTE KAMAE HEAD: LEFT PALM TO RIGHT TEMPLE. (MOVEMENT: NONE. BREATH: IN THROUGH NOSE, RELEASE THROUGH MOUTH.

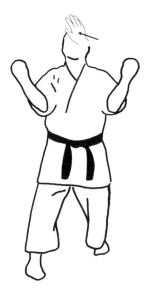

MOROTE KAMAE HEAD: RIGHT PALM TO FOREHEAD. (MOVEMENT: NONE. BREATH: IN THROUGH NOSE, RELEASE THROUGH MOUTH).

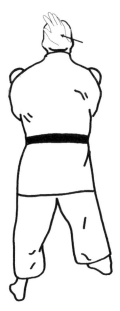

MOROTE KAMAE HEAD: RIGHT PALM TO BACK OF HEAD. (MOVEMENT: NONE. BREATH: IN THROUGH NOSE, RELEASE THROUGH MOUTH).

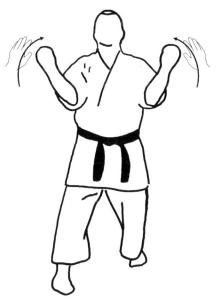

MOROTE KAMAE HANDS: BOTH PALMS PUSHING TOWARD BODY, EQUAL PRESSURE. (MOVEMENT: NONE. BREATH: IN THROUGH NOSE, RELEASE THROUGH MOUTH).

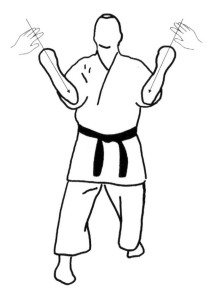

MOROTE KAMAE HANDS: BOTH PALMS TO BOTH HANDS,
DOWNWARD AND EQUAL PRESSURE. (MOVEMENT: NONE.
BREATH: IN THROUGH NOSE, RELEASE THROUGH MOUTH).

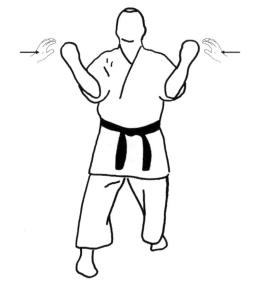

MOROTE KAMAE HANDS: BOTH PALMS TO BOTH HANDS,
INWARD AND EQUAL PRESSURE. (MOVEMENT: NONE.
BREATH: IN THROUGH NOSE, RELEASE THROUGH MOUTH).

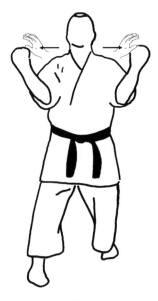

MOROTE KAMAE HANDS: BOTH PALMS TO BOTH HANDS,
OUTWARD AND EQUAL PRESSURE. (MOVEMENT: NONE.
BREATH: IN THROUGH NOSE, RELEASE THROUGH MOUTH).

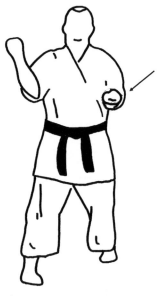

LEFT ARM BACK INTO CHAMBER.
(BREATH: IN THROUGH NOSE).

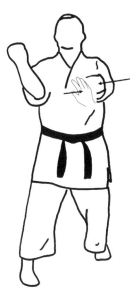

RIGHT PALM TO KNUCKLES OF LEFT FIST, PRESSURE DURING
EXECUTION OF PUNCH. (MOVEMENT: LEFT ARM PUNCH.
BREATH: OUT THROUGH MOUTH).

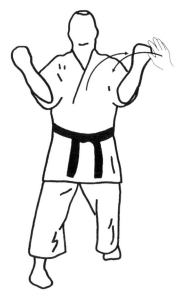

RIGHT PALM GIVING PRESSURE TO OUTSIDE OF LEFT FIST.
(MOVEMENT: RETURN TO CHEST BLOCK. BREATH: IN
THROUGH NOSE).

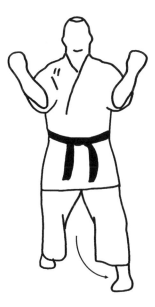

LEFT STEP FORWARD INTO SANCHIN DACHI.
(BREATH: NONE).

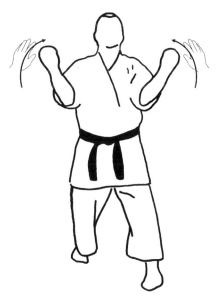

MOROTE KAMAE HANDS: BOTH PALMS PUSHING TOWARD
BODY, EQUAL PRESSURE. (MOVEMENT: NONE. BREATH: IN
THROUGH NOSE, RELEASE THROUGH MOUTH).

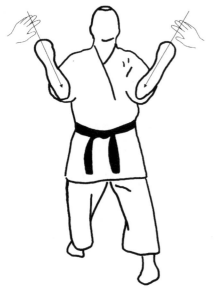

MOROTE KAMAE HANDS: BOTH PALMS TO BOTH HANDS, DOWNWARD AND EQUAL PRESSURE. (MOVEMENT: NONE. BREATH: IN THROUGH NOSE, RELEASE THROUGH MOUTH).

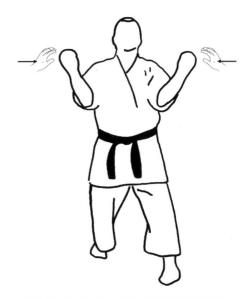

MOROTE KAMAE HANDS: BOTH PALMS TO BOTH HANDS, INWARD AND EQUAL PRESSURE. (MOVEMENT: NONE. BREATH: IN THROUGH NOSE, RELEASE THROUGH MOUTH).

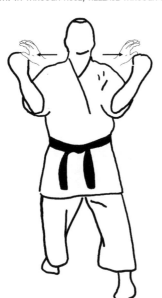

MOROTE KAMAE HANDS: BOTH PALMS TO BOTH HANDS, OUTWARD AND EQUAL PRESSURE. (MOVEMENT: NONE. BREATH: IN THROUGH NOSE, RELEASE THROUGH MOUTH).

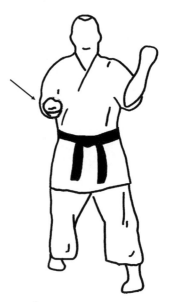

RIGHT ARM BACK INTO CHAMBER. (BREATH: IN THROUGH NOSE).

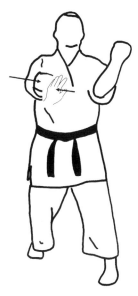

LEFT PALM TO KNUCKLES OF RIGHT FIST, PRESSURE DURING EXECUTION OF PUNCH. (MOVEMENT: RIGHT ARM PUNCH. BREATH: OUT THROUGH MOUTH).

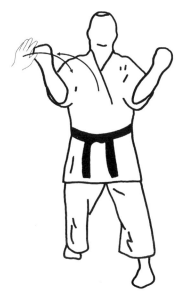

LEFT PALM GIVING PRESSURE TO OUTSIDE OF RIGHT FIST. (MOVEMENT: RETURN TO CHEST BLOCK. BREATH: IN THROUGH NOSE).

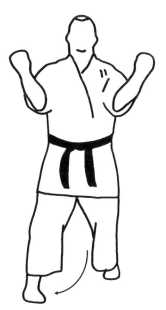

RIGHT STEP FORWARD INTO SANCHIN DACHI. (BREATH: NONE).

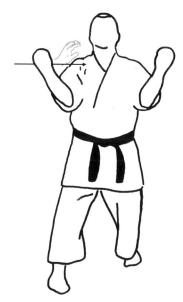

MOROTE KAMAE SHOULDER: LEFT PALM TO RIGHT SHOULDER, PRESSURE TO CENTERLINE. (MOVEMENT: NONE, BREATH: IN THROUGH NOSE, RELEASE THROUGH MOUTH).

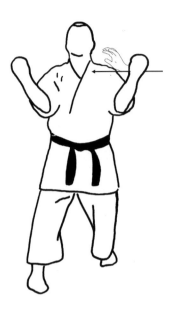

MOROTE KAMAE SHOULDER: RIGHT PALM TO LEFT SHOUL-
DER, PRESSURE TO CENTERLINE. (MOVEMENT: NONE.
BREATH: IN THROUGH NOSE, RELEASE THROUGH MOUTH).

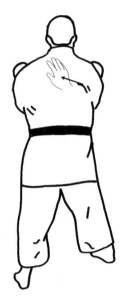

MOROTE KAMAE BACK: RIGHT PALM TO BACK, BETWEEN
SHOULDER BLADES. (MOVEMENT: NONE. BREATH: IN
THROUGH NOSE, RELEASE THROUGH MOUTH).

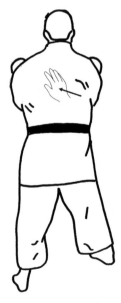

MOROTE KAMAE BACK: RIGHT PALM TO BACK, MID-SPINE.
(MOVEMENT: NONE. BREATH: IN THROUGH NOSE, RELEASE
THROUGH MOUTH).

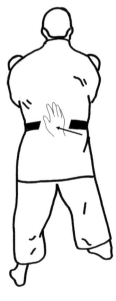

MOROTE KAMAE BACK: RIGHT PALM TO TOP OF SACRUM AND
LAST LUMBAR VERTEBRA. (MOVEMENT: NONE. BREATH: IN
THROUGH NOSE, RELEASE THROUGH MOUTH).

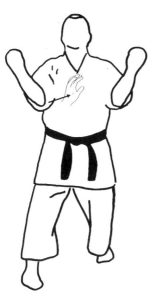

MOROTE KAMAE TORSO: LEFT PALM PUSHING INTO STER-
NUM. (MOVEMENT: NONE. BREATH: IN THROUGH NOSE,
RELEASE THROUGH MOUTH).

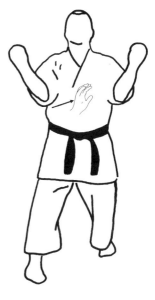

MOROTE KAMAE TORSO: LEFT PALM PUSHING INTO SOLAR
PLEXUS. (MOVEMENT: NONE. BREATH: IN THROUGH NOSE,
RELEASE THROUGH MOUTH).

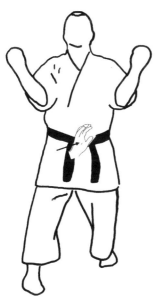

MOROTE KAMAE TORSO: LEFT PALM PUSHING INTO HARA.
(MOVEMENT: NONE. BREATH: IN THROUGH NOSE, RELEASE
THROUGH MOUTH).

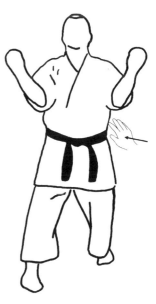

MOROTE KAMAE HIP: RIGHT PALM TO LEFT HIP, PRESSURE
TO CENTERLINE. (MOVEMENT: NONE. BREATH: IN THROUGH
NOSE, RELEASE THROUGH MOUTH).

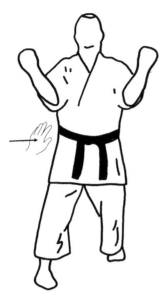

MOROTE KAMAE HIP: LEFT PALM TO RIGHT HIP, PRESSURE TO CENTERLINE. (MOVEMENT: NONE. BREATH: IN THROUGH NOSE, RELEASE THROUGH MOUTH).

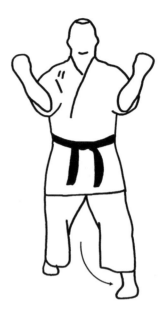

LEFT STEP FORWARD INTO SANCHIN DACHI. (BREATH: NONE).

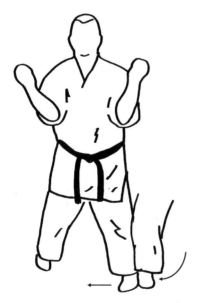

MOROTE KAMAE LOWER LEG: OUTSIDE OF LEFT FOOT TO OUTSIDE OF LEFT FOOT, PRESSURE ON KNEE TOWARD CENTERLINE. (MOVEMENT: NONE. BREATH: IN THROUGH NOSE, RELEASE THROUGH MOUTH).

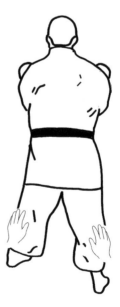

MOROTE KAMAE LOWER LEG: BOTH PALMS TO CALVES FROM REAR, WITH FORWARD AND SLIGHTLY DOWNWARD PRESSURE (MOVEMENT: NONE. BREATH: IN THROUGH NOSE, RELEASE THROUGH MOUTH).

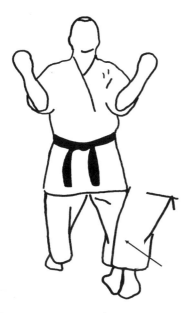

MOROTE KAMAE LOWER LEG: LEFT KNEE TO LEFT KNEE OF FORWARD LEG, BACKWARD PRESSURE (MOVEMENT: NONE. BREATH: IN THROUGH NOSE, RELEASE THROUGH MOUTH).

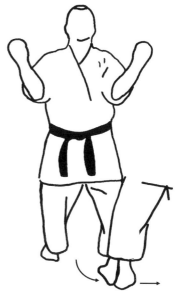

MOROTE KAMAE LOWER LEG: LEFT INSIDE OF FOOT TO LEFT INSIDE OF FOOT, HEEL TO TOE, OUTWARD SWEEPING PRESSURE (MOVEMENT: NONE. BREATH: IN THROUGH NOSE, RELEASE THROUGH MOUTH).

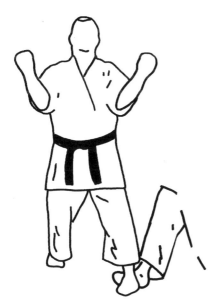

MOROTE KAMAE LOWER LEG: RIGHT INSIDE OF FOOT TO LEFT HEEL, FORWARD SWEEPING PRESSURE (MOVEMENT: NONE. BREATH: IN THROUGH NOSE, RELEASE THROUGH MOUTH).

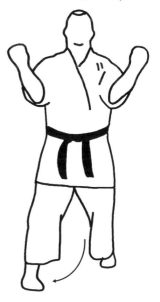

RIGHT STEP FORWARD INTO SANCHIN DACHI. (BREATH: NONE).

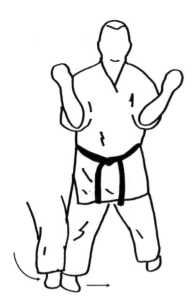

MOROTE KAMAE LOWER LEG: OUTSIDE OF RIGHT FOOT TO OUTSIDE OF RIGHT FOOT, PRESSURE ON KNEE TOWARD CENTERLINE. (MOVEMENT: NONE. BREATH: IN THROUGH NOSE, RELEASE THROUGH MOUTH).

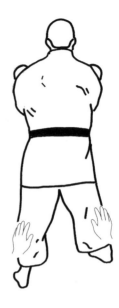

MOROTE KAMAE LOWER LEG: BOTH PALMS TO CALVES FROM REAR, WITH FORWARD AND SLIGHTLY DOWNWARD PRESSURE (MOVEMENT: NONE. BREATH: IN THROUGH NOSE, RELEASE THROUGH MOUTH).

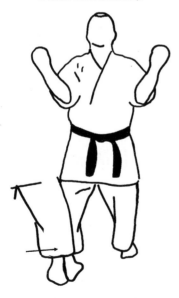

MOROTE KAMAE LOWER LEG: RIGHT KNEE TO RIGHT KNEE OF FORWARD LEG, BACKWARD PRESSURE (MOVEMENT: NONE. BREATH: IN THROUGH NOSE, RELEASE THROUGH MOUTH).

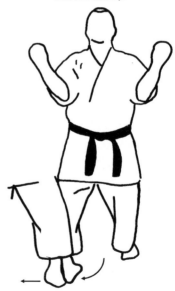

MOROTE KAMAE LOWER LEG: RIGHT INSIDE OF FOOT TO RIGHT INSIDE OF FOOT, HEEL TO TOE, OUTWARD SWEEPING PRESSURE (MOVEMENT: NONE. BREATH: IN THROUGH NOSE, RELEASE THROUGH MOUTH).

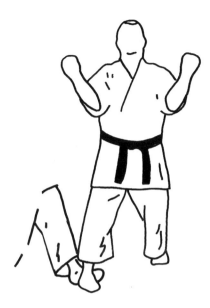

Morote kamae lower leg: Left inside of foot to right heel, forward sweeping pressure (Movement: None. Breath: In through nose, release through mouth).

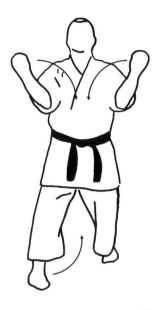

Right step backward into sanchin dachi (Movement: Double chest block. Breath: None).

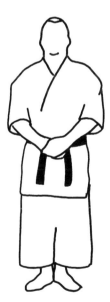

Yoi (Movement: None. Breath: In through nose, release through mouth, deep, half of your maximum capacity).

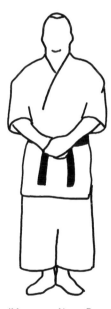

Yoi, breathing (Movement: None. Breath: In through nose, release through mouth, deeper, maximum capacity).

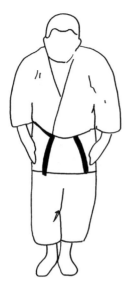

BOW

The order in this description is from the outside inward to the core from the top of the body downward. It is just fine to work from the feet to the head, or just work one section. There is no need to start in one place as the body should be unified and all parts of the body come into play at various levels. Clearly, if one plans to test the entire body, then starting at one end and moving to the other makes sense for order. It is also important to note that if an emphasis needs to be placed on a point not listed because of individual needs move there and test.

What to look for

This is where everything we have discussed in this book comes into play. When testing, it is important to look at the, arms, feet, legs, and so on with an eye toward the nuances that have been discussed. A well-trained eye will be able to understands what needs to be tested, adjusted or reset, and in what degree. It is, thus, a position of responsibility.

It is always best to find someone versed in *sanchin kata* and seek their expertise. However, not having that person at hand is no reason not to practice the *kata* since most practitioners practice other techniques and *kata* unsupervised. *Sanchin kata* should be no different. Do not shy away from your efforts to learn and work with others or by yourself. *Sanchin kata* presents the opportunity to refine a rich variety of techniques, both mental and physical that will have positive benefit far beyond the *kata* itself. It should be understood that *sanchin kata* is about core, core technique, and core understanding. When these core fundamentals are practiced, the benefits to one's karate will be far reaching.

CHAPTER TWENTY-THREE

Implements for Sanchin Kata Training

Keep away from people who try to belittle your ambitions. Small people always do that, but the really great ones make you feel that you too, can become great.

—Mark Twain [55]

Traditional martial arts training implements such as the *makiwara* (punching board) and *chishi* (a leveraged weight) are excellent for honing the techniques essential to the practice of *sanchin kata*. A discussion of both implements follows.

The Makiwara

There are many opinions on the use of the *makiwara* ranging from being an absolute essential to being a device for damaging your body. Like most things in life, moderation and correct use are the cornerstones to benefiting the maximum out of the *makiwara*.

One way to look at the *makiwara* is the same way a former college roommate and pharmacist explained drugs and pharmacology to me, "The difference between a medicine and a poison is often simply the dosage level." This statement applies when using the *makiwara*. The deliberate deforming of the hand, or any part of the body, in the name of training, has no place in martial arts. In fact, it is contrary to its very nature.

Some would argue that the traditional ways from China involved plunging the hands into vessels of sand or rock, and even heated in some instances as well. Maybe so; life expectancy, however, has increased three decades since the 1900s and as a billboard in the Midwest proclaimed as I drove by, "Your body—where you will live the rest of your life!" Simply put, moderation and personal responsibility are required if one hopes to enjoy long-term physical health.

Building a Makiwara

The Okinawan people are well known for their ability to make do with what is at hand. A *makiwara* is an excellent example of that ability because it is an object traditionally built of ready resources. As such, there is no gold standard to the construc-

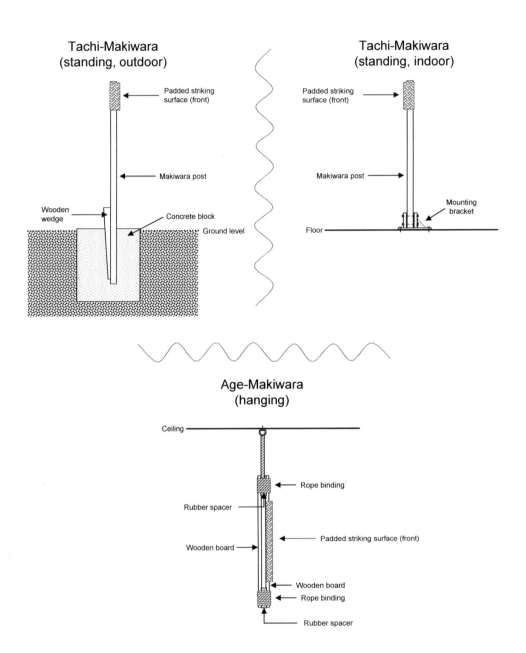

THE *MAKIWARA* (ILLUSTRATION COURTESY OF LAWRENCE A. KANE).

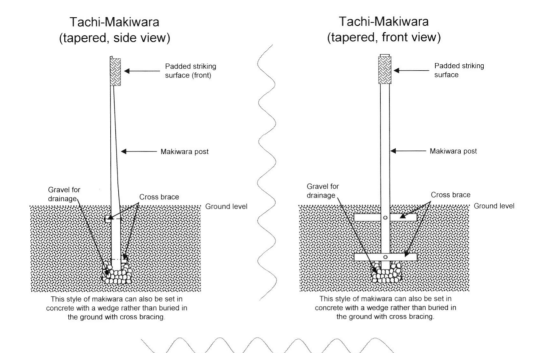

Tachi-Makiwara (tapered, side view)

Padded striking surface (front)

Makiwara post

Gravel for drainage

Cross brace

Ground level

This style of makiwara can also be set in concrete with a wedge rather than buried in the ground with cross bracing.

Tachi-Makiwara (tapered, front view)

Padded striking surface

Makiwara post

Gravel for drainage

Cross brace

Ground level

This style of makiwara can also be set in concrete with a wedge rather than buried in the ground with cross bracing.

Tachi-Makiwara (pole-style)

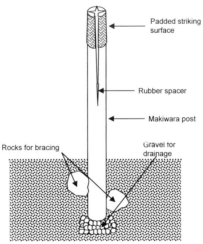

Padded striking surface

Rubber spacer

Makiwara post

Rocks for bracing

Gravel for drainage

This style of makiwara can also be set in concrete rather than buried directly in the ground.

tion of a *makiwara*. They can be mounted in the back yard, set in concrete, screwed to a support beam, or, as I have seen, bolted to the floor in the storage room of a health club. Historically, buried logs in parallel orientation to the upright *makiwara* provided the resistance needed that concrete now provides.

Fundamentally, the vertical board, the *makiwara*, needs to be secured and any means that suit your training environment is fine.

The *makiwara* post itself can be as tall as your chin or as tall as your chest. The choice is yours. The *makiwara* sometimes is made out of trimmed boards, thicker at the bottom of the board and thinner at the top, to give more flexibility. I have also seen them made out of two-inch by six-inch boards with no trimming, three-quarter-inch deep by four inches wide and made of a variety of woods, from pine to oak.

One spring while training in *Sensei* Teruo Chinen's home garden, he put several of us to work building a *makiwara*. It involved digging a hole about two feet deep and eighteen inches wide. A two-by-six board, two inches thick and six inches wide, was held vertical in the hole with a wedge board of the same width and about two-and-a-half feet tall was held in the hole and flush to the *makiwara*. The purpose of the wedge board is to keep the makiwara in place as well as to allow for the replacement of a broken *makiwara* by removing it to extract, and then to wedge a new one back in place. To this hole, we added concrete and held the board and wedge in place until the concrete had set. The bottom line regarding mounting a *makiwara* is that it needs to be secure.

The padding was traditionally made of rice straw because that is what was available. From a traditional, historic standpoint, using such padding creates a classic look. However, it does not take the abuse as well as modern materials. A person can use anything from leather to synthetics to make the striking surface of the *makiwara*. It is important that the surface be blemish free, no bumps, or poor wrapping because these can cause injury.

A *makiwara* needs to flex when it is struck. With no flexibility, a *makiwara* simply becomes a steel pole and damage to your body will result. In the same way that a person who works on their feet all day uses padded matting and shoes to save their joints and back, you need some flexibility in your *makiwara* for all the same reasons.

Large knuckles and calluses are a result, not the objective, of training. The goal of the *makiwara* is training the body to operate in concert, not building big knuckles. Here is a way to look at it. If you were to take the field in a National Football League game, you had all the pads, and a helmet and the other professional football players were unprotected, would you still want to be hit by them? The answer is, "no," you do not want to get hit by them because the football players' fundamental skills, technique, and physical training are what separate them from you, not the gear. Muhammad Ali, Jack Dempsey, and Larry Holmes, as well as other boxing greats did not have enlarged knuckles. Furthermore, boxers wear gloves and still successfully knock out opponents. Again, to underscore the point, success is about technique, not trappings.

Other options

Striking pads, focus mitts, heavy bags, water bags, and other training aids are not direct replacements for the *makiwara*. The reason for this is the *makiwara* gives instant and direct feedback in the form of non-recoiled pressure. As a heavy bag moves away from your fist and swings back when stuck, it takes time to sway from your strike and then return. The *makiwara* gives instant pressure—the harder you hit, the harder it gives pressure back toward you.

Makiwara: Drill 1

Stand in front of your *makiwara* in *sanchin dachi*. Although you will switch sides, begin with your left foot forward. Place your right fist against the *makiwara* at throat level. As always, measurements are done against your own body, so throat level on the *makiwara* is your throat level. Without leaning into the *makiwara*, shift slightly forward to bend the *makiwara* just enough so you feel a firm pressure. While holding this position, audit your structure, starting with your footing and then moving up your body. As you do this, be attentive to the muscles you are using. The less contraction of muscle prior to contact, the more explosive the muscles are upon contact. In a effort to promote balance in your body, be sure and switch sides to right foot forward, left-hand punch, and perform the structure audit again.

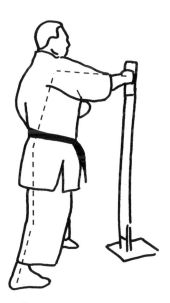

HOLDING BEND IN *MAKIWARA* IN ORDER TO AUDIT BODY STRUCTURE.

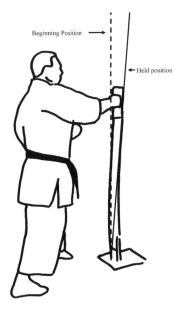

Beginning Position →

← Held position

STRIKING *MAKIWARA*.

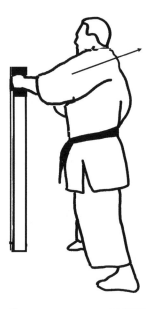

STRIKING *MAKIWARA* AND ALLOWING
RECOIL INTO BODY VIA SHOULDER.

Makiwara: Drill 2

This drill focuses on the moment after the strike, to build an understanding of the sensation of the rebound action of the *makiwara*. Again, stand in *sanchin dachi* as described in the previous drill and strike the *makiwara*. Now, hold the strike. Do not allow the *makiwara* to move back to its original position even slightly. Once the initial bounce-back from the strike has taken place in the *makiwara,* you can release the strike and begin again. Go slowly as you start training. Just like the *kata,* the slower you go the better you can absorb what is taking place. Do not advance too quickly either. Trying to be fast too soon will rob you of the experience of the rebound from the *makiwara.* This sensation needs to be felt in order to

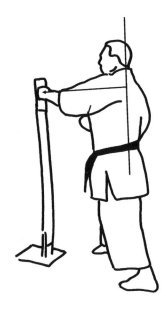

STRIKING *MAKIWARA* AND NOT ALLOWING RECOIL.

be fully understood. As with any training procedure, as the practitioner becomes familiar with the timing, it is possible to increase speed without sacrificing technique.

This drill helps you keep your form and muscle structure in proper placement. This drill will result in the practitioner hitting harder and stronger in a brief amount of training time. Oddly enough the better the practitioner the less results will be seen. Conversely, the less skilled the practitioner is in the beginning, the greater the improvement and in less time.

Makiwara: Drill 3

This drill should not be undertaken without extensive practice and considerations of your physical strength. Again, starting in *sanchin dachi*, strike the *makiwara* with a fore fist, or *seiken*. After becoming familiar with the distance necessary to connect properly with the *makiwara*, close your eyes and continue striking the *makiwara*, slowly at first. If you are using a simple leather-covered *makiwara*, that is, with little padding, you need to be extra cautious. A damaged hand takes a very long time to heal and will add a substantial amount of downtime to your training.

This drill will bring confidence to your striking without needing to see the punch.

The Chishi

The *chishi*, a leveraged weight, traditionally consisted of a stone mounted on the end of a stick. Today it is often concrete or plaster poured around a stick. The use of the *chishi* is fairly direct; it is swung and lifted in various ways to build muscle strength and technique, adjusting the desired weight by moving the hands up and down on the handle.

Building a Chishi

Like the *makiwara,* there are many ways and no exclusive "right way" to build a *chishi*. The following, however, is the easiest. A plastic tub, one used for margarine, is a good size to begin with. You will also need some quick-setting concrete mix, about four nails or screws, and a

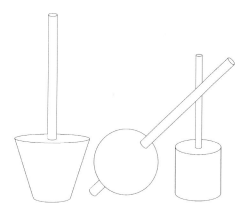

THE *CHISHI*.

piece of wooden curtain rod about two feet in length. At the end of the curtain rod, drive the nails or screws in the wood. These will serve to anchor the wood into the concrete. Place the handle into the plastic tub and support the handle in a vertical position any way you choose. Pour the mixed concrete into the tub and leave overnight. In the morning, cut the tub away and begin training.

Chishi: Drill 1

When executing this *chishi* drill, it is important to remember this is not a traditional Western weightlifting drill. It is instead based on velocity and focus.

Standing in *sanchin dachi* with the right foot forward, grasp the *chishi* by the handle with your little finger on the stone

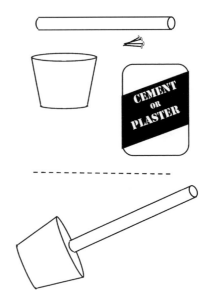

MATERIALS NEEDED TO BUILD A *CHISHI*: STICK, NAILS, QUIKRETE™ OR PLASTER.

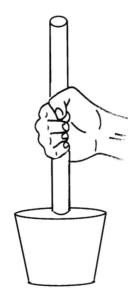

GRIPPING *CHISHI* IN LOWER BLOCK LITTLE FINGER TO WEIGHT SIDE.

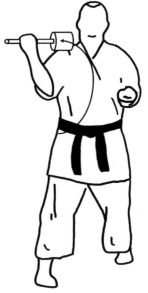

SNAPPING *CHISHI* INTO CHEST BLOCK POSITION.

side and the thumb riding close to the end of the handle. Hold the *chishi* at arm's length in a down-block position (*gedan uke*).

With a snapping motion, bring the *chishi* up into a chest block (*chudan uke*). The *chishi* needs to be held horizontal to the floor. The final gripping and rotation of the hand holding the *chishi* should bring the stone closer to the chest.

The opposite arm while in chamber should mimic the same flinch of tension of the arm holding the *chishi*. This mimicking of one side of the body by the other helps in unifying the body.

Chishi Drill 2

The point of this drill is to control the *chishi* while using the correct muscles for performing *sanchin kata*. The focus should be on:

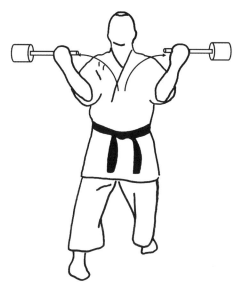

Morote kamae (double chest block) with *chishi* in both hands (Movement: Right step forward to *sanchin dachi*. Breath: Hold, release through mouth; In and out, shallow).

1. Architecture. It is important to keep the architecture of *sanchin kata* in place. The bones need to be aligned as described in earlier chapters and remain this way during the entire *kata*. Be especially attentive to the elbows to ensure they stay close to the body and do not hunch your back as you become tired.

2. Muscle control. The pectoral, and latissimus, tension and release are of a prime concern during this drill.

Now, perform *sanchin kata* with the *chishi* in your hands the entire time. Because the *kata* should be done at a slow pace, do this exercise slowly as if doing Western weightlifting. Once you have completed the *kata* with the *chishi*, do it again immediately afterward without the *chishi* for a total of two repetitions.

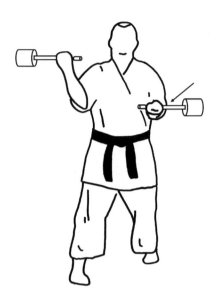

SANCHIN KATA PULL BACK TO CHAMBER IN PREPARATION FOR STRIKE (MOVEMENT: LEFT ARM BACK TO CHAMBER. BREATH: IN THROUGH NOSE; IN AND OUT, SHALLOW).

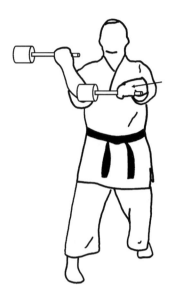

STRIKING WITH *CHISHI* IN HAND (MOVEMENT: LEFT PUNCH. BREATH: OUT THROUGH MOUTH; IN AND OUT, SHALLOW).

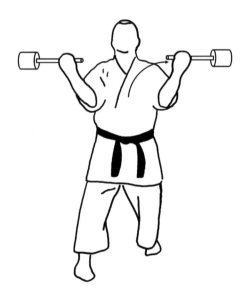

SANCHIN KATA PUNCH RETURNED TO *MOROTE KAMAE* (DOUBLE CHEST BLOCK) (MOVEMENT: RIGHT STEP FORWARD TO *SANCHIN DACHI*. BREATH: HOLD, RELEASE THROUGH MOUTH; IN AND OUT, SHALLOW).

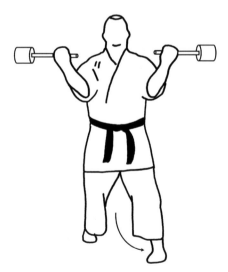

STEP FORWARD WITH LEFT FOOT (MOVEMENT: STEP FORWARD LEFT FOOT. BREATH: HOLD; IN AND OUT, SHALLOW).

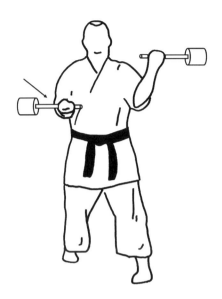

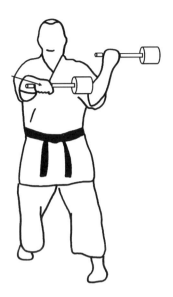

SANCHIN KATA PULL BACK TO CHAMBER IN PREPARATION FOR STRIKE (MOVEMENT: PULL RIGHT ARM BACK TO CHAMBER. BREATH: IN THROUGH NOSE; IN AND OUT, SHALLOW)

STRIKING WITH *CHISHI* IN HAND (MOVEMENT: RIGHT PUNCH TO CENTERLINE. BREATH: OUT THROUGH MOUTH; IN AND OUT, SHALLOW).

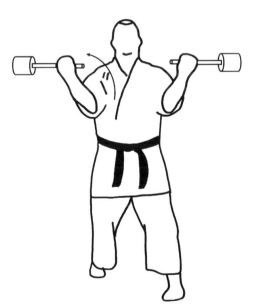

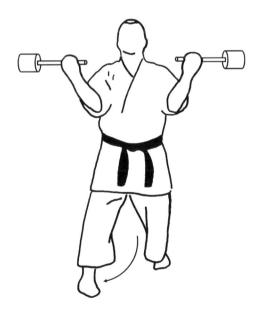

SANCHIN KATA PUNCH RETURNED TO *MOROTE KAMAE* (DOUBLE CHEST BLOCK) (MOVEMENT: STEP FORWARD LEFT FOOT. BREATH: HOLD; IN AND OUT, SHALLOW).

STEP FORWARD WITH RIGHT FOOT (MOVEMENT: RIGHT STEP FORWARD TO *SANCHIN DACHI*. BREATH: HOLD, RELEASE THROUGH MOUTH; IN AND OUT, SHALLOW).

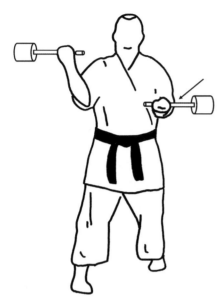

SANCHIN KATA PULL BACK TO CHAMBER IN PREPARATION FOR
STRIKE (MOVEMENT: LEFT ARM BACK TO CHAMBER. BREATH:
IN THROUGH NOSE; IN AND OUT, SHALLOW).

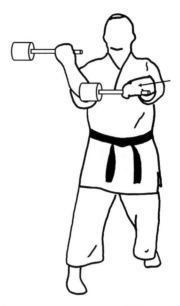

STRIKING WITH *CHISHI* IN HAND (MOVEMENT: LEFT PUNCH.
BREATH: OUT THROUGH MOUTH; IN AND OUT, SHALLOW).

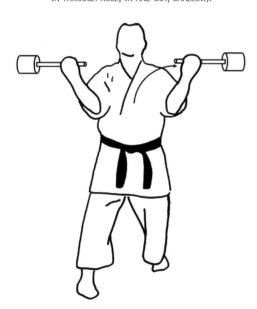

SANCHIN KATA PUNCH RETURNED TO *MOROTE KAMAE* (DOU-
BLE CHEST BLOCK) (MOVEMENT: RIGHT STEP FORWARD TO
SANCHIN DACHI. BREATH: HOLD, RELEASE THROUGH
MOUTH; IN AND OUT, SHALLOW).

Chishi: Drill 3

Once again standing in *sanchin dachi*, grip the bottom of the *chishi* handle and hold the *chishi* stone upward at arm's length chest high in front of yourself in a vertical position. With the *chishi* stone held high, begin to move the stone in a circle using your hand to generate the motion. The *chishi* should move in a circle about the size of a dinner plate. Keep your elbow in and deltoid (shoulder) muscle relaxed. Reversing the motion is also part of the drill. No certain number of repetitions is required, nor is a particular circle size mandated for the movement of the *chishi*. However, it is better to use a lighter weight with more repetitions instead of fewer done with a heavier weight.

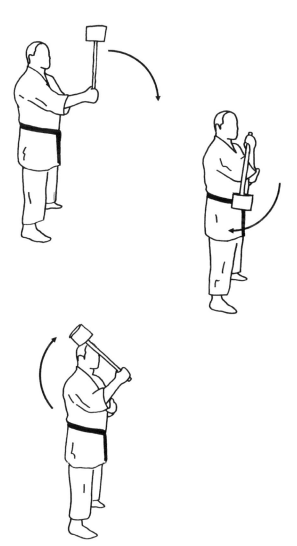

CHISHI HELD IN FRONT AT ARM'S LENGTH AND MOVED IN CIRCULAR MOTION.

CHAPTER TWENTY-FOUR

Breathing

Nature, to be commanded, must be obeyed.

—*Sir Francis Bacon* [56]

Breathing is the most essential part of a human being's existence. Depending on the circumstances, you can go without food for a month, water for three days, and air maybe a minute and a half. However, because breathing is so basic to our existence, its importance to the practice of martial arts is rarely considered. However, the proper execution of *sanchin kata* requires a mastery of a specialized form of breathing as well as storage of air within the body. Among the core teachings embedded in the *kata* are the benefits of controlled breathing techniques to the vascular system and to lung capacity, as well as to attaining a strong body architecture that allows one to withstand blows with ease.

It is commonly known that on a daily basis, people typically use only a small portion of their lung capacity. The expansion and depth that are characteristic of *sanchin kata* breathing allow the lungs to be much more completely filled, to great and varied benefit.

The alveoli are the tiny sac-like spaces at the end of the bronchioles in the lungs, are where carbon dioxide and oxygen are exchanged. Oxygen moves from the alveoli (high oxygen concentration) to the blood (lower oxygen concentration). The oxygen first dissolves in the fluid in the interstitial tissues and diffuses into the blood. Oxygen binds to hemoglobin in the red blood cells, which allows a greater amount of oxygen to be transported by the blood. Red blood cells are ready and quick to pick up as much available oxygen as possible. Because of this efficiency, the actual respiratory drive is the expulsion of the carbon dioxide, not pulling in oxygen. It has been suggested that while breathing creates pressure in the lungs to allow better oxygen update, this is not the biological function.

The benefits of *sanchin kata* breathing, called "*ibuki* breathing," are varied. From a mechanical standpoint, it aids in locking down the torso, bringing the ribs, shoulders, back, and abdomen to a taut readiness needed to deliver power and withstand blows. The architecture of the body must be in place prior to beginning the *ibuki* breathing for it to be effective. In addition, *ibuki* breathing places the focus of the breath in the belly helping anchor the body and the mind, and exercises the vascular system, strengthening both lungs and diaphragm. Below is a discussion of the elements of *ibuki* breathing.

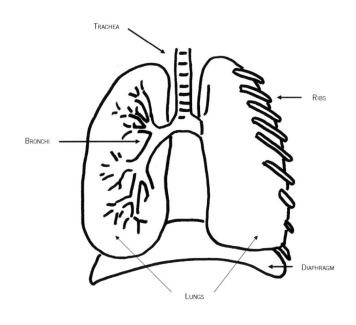

THE LUNGS.

The Inhale

The inhale is done through the nose and moves through the front of the skull to the top of the head, then to the back of the head and down the back through the spine. Hitting the base of the sacrum, the breath moves to the center of the body. This area is called many things, the *hara*, root (or *muladhara*), *chakra*, or *tanden*. No matter the term, it is all the same place and all the same thing.

To assist the practitioner's efforts in moving the breath through the body, the following imagery is recommended. As you breathe in, imagine the movement of the breath as follows: Once the breath has moved to the center of your body, the *hara*, make the breath swirl around itself several times. There is no mandated number of rotations of the breath or speed at which it should rotate. One of my instructors used to say, "It is like winding thread on a spool."

The Exhale

The exhale begins by unwinding the spool of your breath. This unwinding is done a little faster than the winding so you will want to adhere to a timing ratio of 5:7, described below. In the same way that a weightlifter exerts force when pushing the weight away from their body, you need to do the same, albeit with less external force. The breath exits straight up the core of the body rising quickly to the throat where a slight restriction of the breath takes place before being expelled through the mouth.

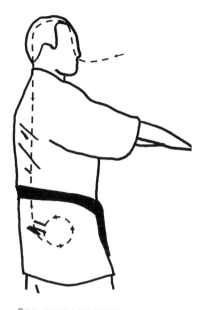 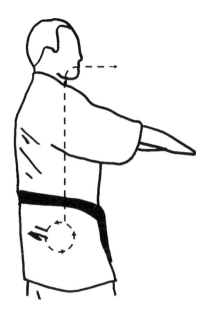

SIDE VIEW OF BODY SHOWING
PATH OF BREATH DURING INHALE.

SIDE VIEW OF BODY SHOWING PATH
OF BREATH DURING EXHALE.

Move your breath in a non-stop circular motion. Once the activity of drawing a breath is begun, the breath is not complete until the breath is exhaled. One way to look at this is the *Yin*, the female is the inhale, and the *Yang*, the male, is the exhale, together making a whole, a complete circle.

The 5:7 Ratio

A complete breath, a full inhale and exhale, is done to a 5:7 ratio of five seconds for an inhale and seven seconds for an exhale. The ratio is the foundation not the number, so doing *sanchin kata* at a 3:5 breath ratio is fine as well as a larger ratio. It is all right to vary your training; however, always bring the training back to the center of the 5:7 ratio. Learn the 5:7 ratio—experiment on your own.

Breath Restriction

Bulging neck veins, tense muscles, and demonic hissing are not part of *sanchin kata*

Much is made of restricting the breath while doing *sanchin kata*. Again, the rule of moderation applies. Restricting the breath too much during the performance of the *kata* can result in escalated blood pressure, throat irritation, or headaches. It should be noted that while there are also rumors that to practice *sanchin kata* in this way leads to hemorrhoids or even premature death. No significant medical study has been done to either substantiate or put to an end to these claims.

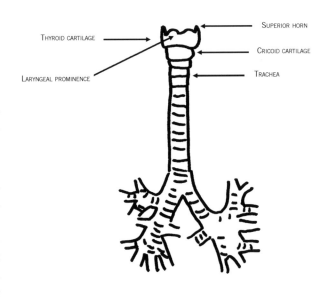

THE TRACHEA.

The breath should be restricted because of the head position upon the neck. When cervical vertebra #1 is pulled into position, the trachea and esophagus are also moved backward causing a constriction. This constriction results in the signature sound of *sanchin kata*, a kind of hissing sound, the same as can often be heard from a sleeping person lying on their back. It is not labored, nor forced; it is simply a restricted airway. This restriction is credited with creating pressure in the lungs, forcing more oxygen into the alveoli of the lungs. Again, this is speculation. In modern athletics, the use of "blood packing," actually increasing the volume of blood in the body through transfusion of an athlete's previously stored blood back into their body, is used to increase performance. Blood packing involves increasing the volume of blood in the body to aid in increasing uptake of, not exposure to, oxygen. This seems to indicate that creating pressure in the lungs to increase oxygen absorption is not the true goal but perhaps is a minor side benefit.

Another element of restricted breathing is the placement of the tongue. Often the ideal placement is described as being on the roof of the mouth; however, that is not quite the target. Determining the placement for the tongue is best done by putting the tip against your front two teeth, and then slightly adjusting it by pulling backward until the tongue sits on the ridge of the gums.

From a physiological standpoint, *ibuki* breathing provides an excellent exercise for the vascular system. Oftentimes we do not use the full capacity of our lungs or employ our diaphragm's full range of motion. It would be foolish to call upon an atrophied system, in this case the lungs, to help us in a time of crisis or combat. Thus, for its physiological benefits alone, *ibuki* breathing makes inherent sense.

CHAPTER TWENTY-FIVE

Turning

The obstacle is the path.

—Zen Proverb

There are two turns in *sanchin kata*. They are both one-hundred-and-eighty-degree counterclockwise turns made by stepping over the left foot with the right foot. When stepping, the right foot crosses over the left foot in an equal amount of distance as it left behind. If the step is not made with the same distance, the stance upon completing the turn is not correct and is too narrow. Whatever the distance between the two feet at the beginning of the step-over into *bensoku dachi*, the same distance must be recreated on the opposite side of the left foot.

To avoid another alignment issue, the stepping foot stays on the same line on which it originated. Failing to do so will result in a shallow stance, which does not allow for good transference of energy.

To execute the turn such that it results in a properly balanced and equal stance at its completion, the body must drop by bending the knees slightly. As the turn is completed, the body pops up via the knees, providing a strong rotation and strong anchored block. This slight thrust or pop upward provides inertia in a vertical plane creating a brief moment of heavier false gravity and giving the practitioner more mass. This motion forces the practitioner upward and into the opponent without leaning and sacrificing balance.*

Keeping the body erect, straight up and down when turning is critical to keeping balance. Bending forward at the waist and turning gives the sensation of generating power from centrifugal force but in fact is just a swinging body. A swinging body is not in control of itself. A swing could be equated to a leap into the air. Once an athlete has left the ground, there is no change in the trajectory until contact with the ground is again made.[57] A swinging body is similar in that the body is sent into motion and great effort is required to stop its momentum prior to completion of the technique. Be aware that swinging gives the sensation of power but it is deceptive and off balance.

---

* Newton's First Law of Motion: Every object in a state of uniform motion tends to remain in that state of motion unless an external force is applied to it.

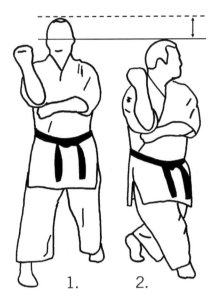

SANCHIN KATA TURN IN PROCESS SHOWING
PROPER HEIGHT THROUGHOUT MOVEMENT.

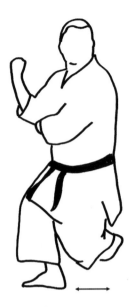

SANCHIN KATA DEPTH OF STEP DURING TURNING MOVEMENT.

Inertia on a Vertical Plane: Test It 1

Simply stand on a scale in your bathroom or health club. Check your weight. Now, bend your knees slightly and thrust upward, and check your weight again. You will notice the reading on the scale will be slightly higher in this position, demonstrating your ability to be heavier for a brief moment.

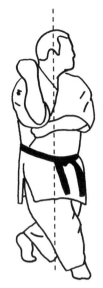

SANCHIN KATA WHILE DOING *BENSOKU DACHI* SHOWING CORRECT POSTURE.

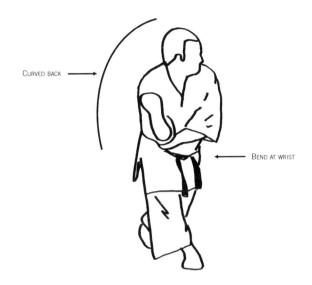

SANCHIN KATA WHILE DOING *BENSOKU DACHI* SHOWING INCORRECT POSTURE WITH BEND AT WAIST.

CHAPTER TWENTY-SIX

The Kata

Nothing will work unless you do.

—*Maya Angelou* [58]

This chapter shows a pattern for *sanchin kata*. As discussed earlier, there are several patterns of *sanchin kata*. The pattern is generally a preference of the instructor and is often directly aligned with what their teacher taught them in respect to the *kata*. No pattern is inherently superior to another. The key lies in the techniques that build the pattern, the understanding of those techniques and their application.

This pattern is a long version and is attributed to Kanryo Higashionna. It is often referred to as the Higashionna version of *sanchin kata*.

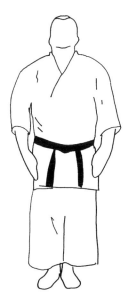

MOVEMENT: NONE
BREATH: IN AND OUT, SHALLOW,

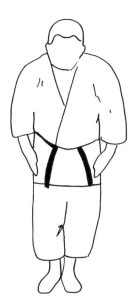

MOVEMENT: BOW
BREATH: NONE.

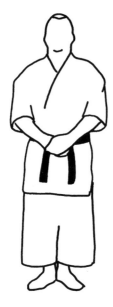

MOVEMENT: NONE
BREATH: IN AND OUT, SHALLOW.

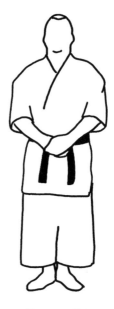

MOVEMENT: NONE
BREATH: IN AND OUT, DEEPER, ONE HALF OF
YOUR MAXIMUM CAPACITY.

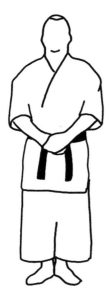

MOVEMENT: NONE
BREATH: IN AND OUT,
DEEPER, MAXIMUM CAPACITY.

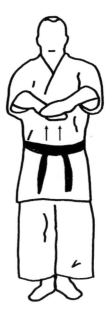

MOVEMENT: RIGHT STEP FORWARD TO SANCHIN DACHI
BREATH: IN THROUGH NOSE.

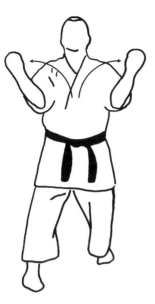

MOVEMENT: RIGHT STEP FORWARD TO SANCHIN DACHI
BREATH: HOLD, RELEASE THROUGH MOUTH.

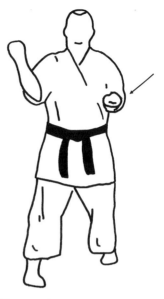

MOVEMENT: LEFT ARM BACK TO CHAMBER
BREATH: IN THROUGH NOSE.

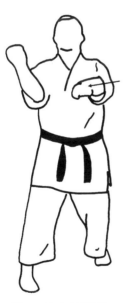

MOVEMENT: LEFT PUNCH
BREATH: OUT THROUGH MOUTH.

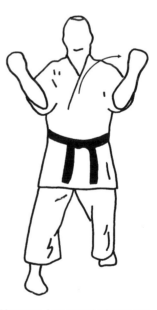

MOVEMENT: LEFT ARM TO CHEST BLOCK
BREATH: IN THROUGH NOSE

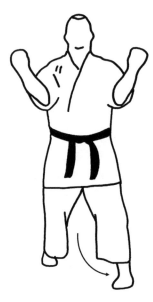

MOVEMENT: STEP FORWARD LEFT FOOT
BREATH: HOLD.

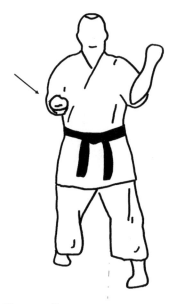

MOVEMENT: PULL RIGHT ARM BACK TO CHAMBER
BREATH: IN THROUGH NOSE.

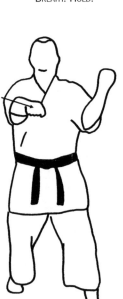

MOVEMENT: RIGHT PUNCH TO CENTERLINE
BREATH: OUT THROUGH MOUTH.

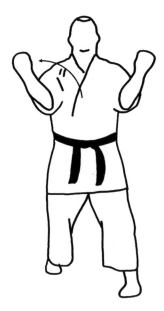

MOVEMENT: RIGHT ARM TO CHEST BLOCK
BREATH: IN THROUGH NOSE.

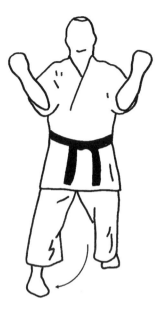

MOVEMENT: STEP FORWARD RIGHT FOOT
BREATH: HOLD.

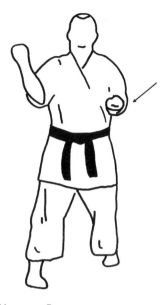

MOVEMENT: PULL LEFT ARM BACK TO CHAMBER
BREATH: IN THROUGH NOSE.

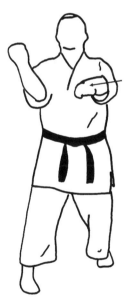

MOVEMENT: LEFT PUNCH TO CENTERLINE
BREATH: OUT THROUGH MOUTH.

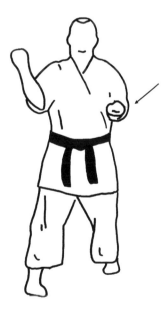

MOVEMENT: LEFT ARM BACK TO CHAMBER
BREATH: IN THROUGH NOSE.

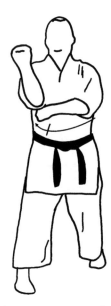

MOVEMENT: LEFT ARM MOVES ACROSS / PALM DOWN
BREATH: HOLD.

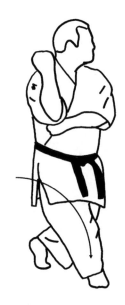

MOVEMENT: RIGHT FOOT STEPS ACROSS
BREATH: HOLD.

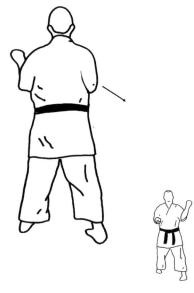

MOVEMENT: RIGHT ARM BACK TO CHAMBER
BREATH: IN THROUGH NOSE.

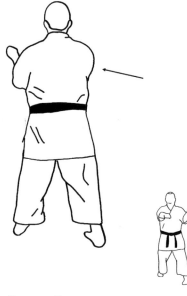

MOVEMENT: RIGHT PUNCH TO CENTERLINE
BREATH: OUT THROUGH MOUTH.

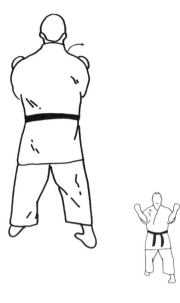

MOVEMENT: RIGHT ARM TO CHEST BLOCK
BREATH: IN THROUGH NOSE.

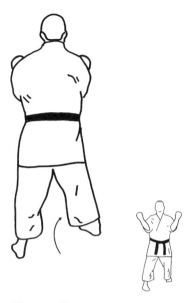

MOVEMENT: STEP FORWARD RIGHT FOOT
BREATH: HOLD.

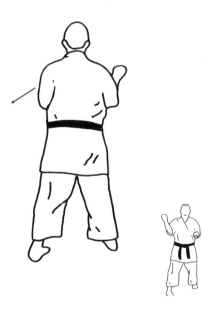

MOVEMENT: PULL LEFT ARM BACK TO CHAMBER
BREATH: IN THROUGH NOSE.

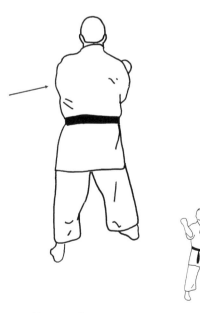

MOVEMENT: LEFT PUNCH TO CENTERLINE
BREATH: OUT THROUGH MOUTH.

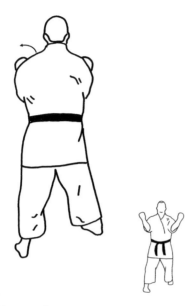

MOVEMENT: LEFT ARM TO CHEST BLOCK
BREATH: IN THROUGH NOSE.

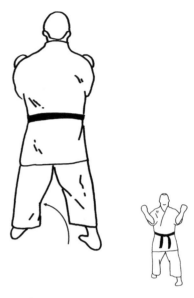

MOVEMENT: LEFT STEP FORWARD TO SANCHIN DACHI
BREATH: HOLD.

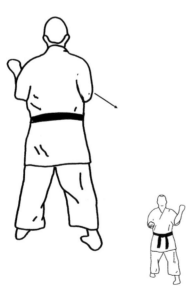

MOVEMENT: PULL RIGHT ARM BACK TO CHAMBER
BREATH: IN THROUGH NOSE.

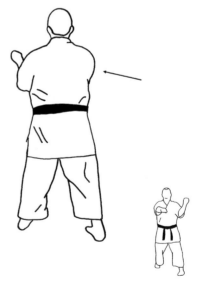

MOVEMENT: RIGHT PUNCH TO CENTERLINE
BREATH: OUT THROUGH MOUTH.

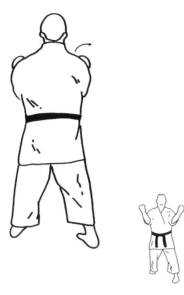

MOVEMENT: RIGHT ARM TO CHEST BLOCK
BREATH: IN THROUGH NOSE.

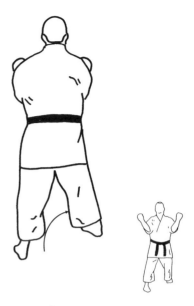

MOVEMENT: STEP FORWARD RIGHT FOOT
BREATH: HOLD.

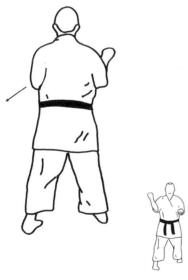

MOVEMENT: PULL LEFT ARM BACK TO CHAMBER
BREATH: IN THROUGH NOSE.

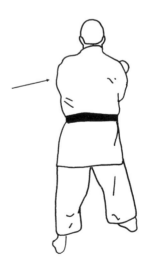

MOVEMENT: LEFT PUNCH TO CENTERLINE
BREATH: OUT THROUGH MOUTH.

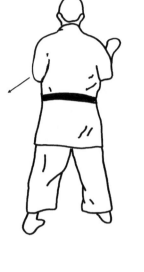
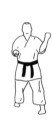

MOVEMENT: PULL LEFT ARM BACK TO CHAMBER
BREATH: IN THROUGH NOSE

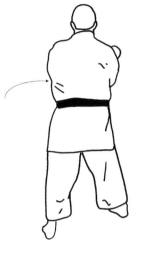
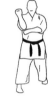

MOVEMENT: LEFT ARM MOVES ACROSS / PALM DOWN
BREATH: HOLD

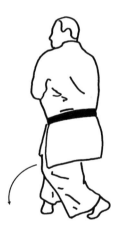
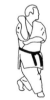

MOVEMENT: RIGHT FOOT STEPS ACROSS
BREATH: HOLD.

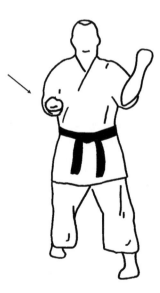

MOVEMENT: RIGHT ARM BACK TO CHAMBER
BREATH: IN THROUGH NOSE.

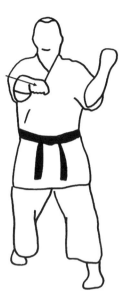

MOVEMENT: RIGHT PUNCH TO CENTERLINE
BREATH: OUT THROUGH MOUTH.

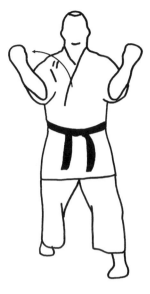

MOVEMENT: RIGHT ARM TO CHEST BLOCK
BREATH: IN THROUGH NOSE.

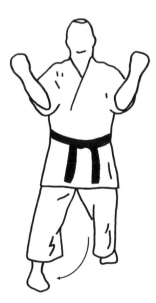

MOVEMENT: STEP FORWARD RIGHT FOOT
BREATH: HOLD.

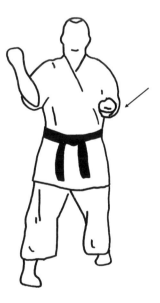

MOVEMENT: PULL LEFT ARM BACK TO CHAMBER
BREATH: IN THROUGH NOSE.

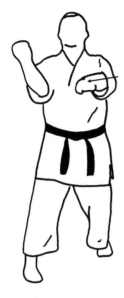

MOVEMENT: LEFT PUNCH TO CENTERLINE
BREATH: OUT THROUGH MOUTH.

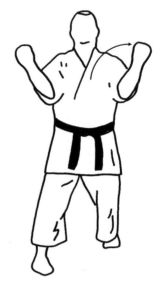

MOVEMENT: LEFT ARM TO CHEST BLOCK
BREATH: IN THROUGH NOSE.

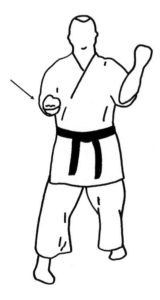

MOVEMENT: PULL RIGHT ARM BACK TO CHAMBER
BREATH: IN THROUGH NOSE.

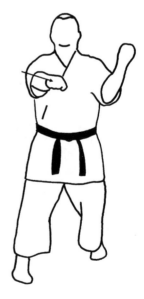

MOVEMENT: RIGHT PUNCH TO CENTERLINE
BREATH: OUT THROUGH MOUTH.

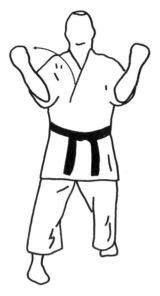

MOVEMENT: RIGHT ARM TO CHEST BLOCK
BREATH: IN THROUGH NOSE.

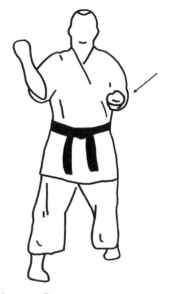

MOVEMENT: PULL LEFT ARM BACK TO CHAMBER
BREATH: IN THROUGH NOSE.

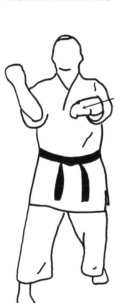

MOVEMENT: LEFT PUNCH TO CENTERLINE
BREATH: OUT THROUGH MOUTH.

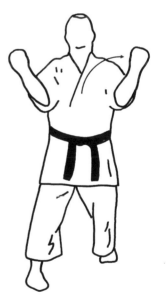

MOVEMENT: LEFT ARM TO CHEST BLOCK
BREATH: IN THROUGH NOSE.

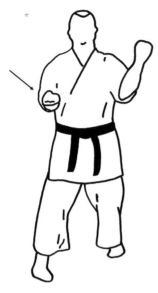

MOVEMENT: NO STEP, PULL RIGHT ARM BACK TO CHAMBER
BREATH: IN THROUGH NOSE.

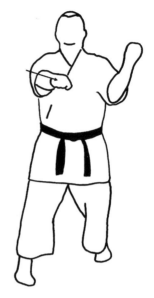

MOVEMENT: RIGHT PUNCH TO CENTERLINE
BREATH: OUT THROUGH MOUTH.

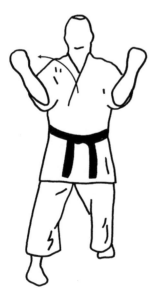

MOVEMENT: RIGHT ARM TO CHEST BLOCK
BREATH: IN THROUGH NOSE.

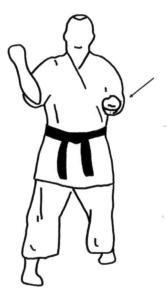

MOVEMENT: PULL LEFT ARM BACK TO CHAMBER
BREATH: IN THROUGH NOSE.

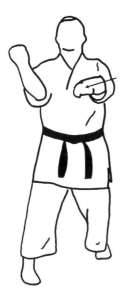

MOVEMENT: LEFT PUNCH TO CENTER LINE
BREATH: OUT THROUGH NOSE.

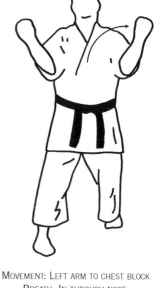

MOVEMENT: LEFT ARM TO CHEST BLOCK
BREATH: IN THROUGH NOSE.

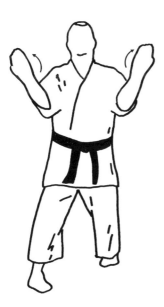

MOVEMENT: OPEN HANDS IN CHEST BLOCK POSITION
BREATH: OUT THROUGH MOUTH

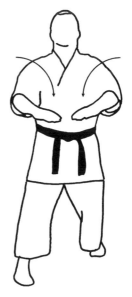

MOVEMENT: PRESS BOTH HANDS DOWNWARD
BREATH: OUT THROUGH MOUTH.

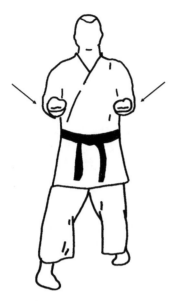

MOVEMENT: BOTH HANDS PULLED BACK TO CHAMBER
BREATH: IN THROUGH NOSE.

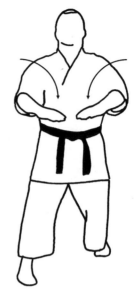

MOVEMENT: PRESS BOTH HANDS DOWNWARD
BREATH: OUT THROUGH MOUTH.

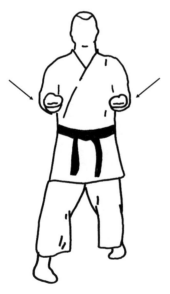

MOVEMENT: BOTH HANDS PULLED BACK TO CHAMBER
BREATH: IN THROUGH NOSE.

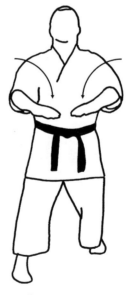

MOVEMENT: PRESS BOTH HANDS DOWNWARD
BREATH: OUT THROUGH MOUTH.

Chapter Twenty-Six: The Kata   163

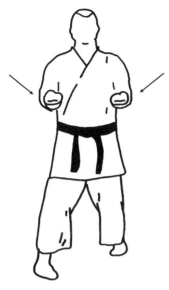

MOVEMENT: BOTH HANDS PULLED BACK TO CHAMBER
BREATH: IN THROUGH NOSE.

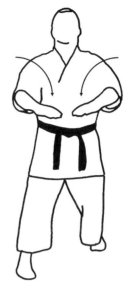

MOVEMENT: PRESS BOTH HANDS DOWNWARD
BREATH: OUT THROUGH MOUTH.

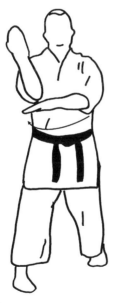

MOVEMENT: LEFT HAND UNDER RIGHT ELBOW PALM DOWN
BREATH: IN THROUGH NOSE.

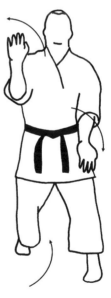

MOVEMENT: MUWASHI UKE, WRAPPING BLOCK
BREATH: IN THROUGH NOSE

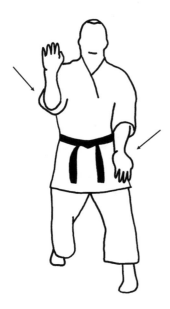

MOVEMENT: SET BOTH HANDS AND ELBOWS
BREATH: OUT THROUGH MOUTH.

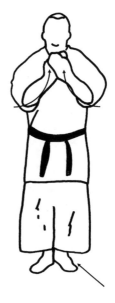

MOVEMENT: BOTH HANDS UP
BREATH: IN THROUGH NOSE.

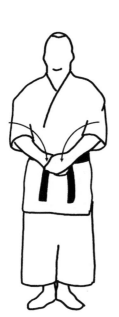

MOVEMENT: NONE
BREATH: OUT THROUGH THE MOUTH.

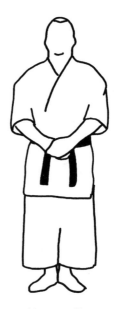

MOVEMENT: NONE
BREATH: OUT THROUGH THE MOUTH.

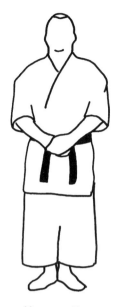

MOVEMENT: NONE
BREATH: OUT THROUGH THE MOUTH.

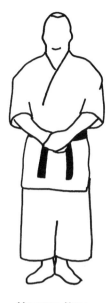

MOVEMENT: NONE
BREATH: IN AND OUT, SHALLOW.

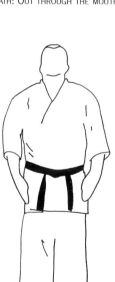

MOVEMENT: NONE
BREATH: IN AND OUT, SHALLOW.

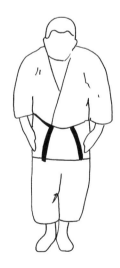

MOVEMENT: BOW
BREATH: NONE.

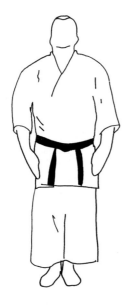

MOVEMENT: NONE
BREATH: IN AND OUT, SHALLOW.

Conclusion

If you think education is expensive, try ignorance.

—*Derek Bok (1930-), Harvard University President* [59]

Sanchin kata is an elemental form that transmits principles of combat, physical health, and mental well-being. It has been changed and molded by those who have taught and studied the form. The common threads that bind all forms and practitioners of *sanchin kata* are breath, stance, and movement—the breath, deep and made with the diaphragm; the stance, one of strength yet flexibility; and movement of the body, the extremities and the core as well.

Sanchin kata offers benefits to the practitioner similar to any physical activity done prudently and with the goal of good health in mind. For example, reduction in stress is one of many benefits. If the body has less stress then a person can devote their energies to the more important aspects of life, instead of having to deal with such things as fighting disease, which is often a side effect of stress. Another example would be the slow movement with synchronized, or timed, breathing that can contribute to a sense of well being. This practice and its benefits are known to yoga practitioners, weightlifters, and many in between these two ends of the spectrum. It also can be noted that because the practice of *sanchin kata* carries no religious beliefs, it can be adapted to a person's training without prejudice. Many practitioners report a calm state of mind and an increased vitality post practice, both of which of course are highly desirable outcomes.

Sanchin kata is a most complete *kata*—simple, yet complex; multifaceted yet clear. For the practitioner that is ready and willing to let the *kata* speak to them, its surface value benefits as well as its deeper mysteries will present new insights, challenges, and joys for a lifetime of training.

Notes

1. (Sarah) Margaret Fuller (1810–1850) was a journalist for the New York Tribune and women's rights activist.
2. Charles Francis Adams (1807–1886, Boston), the son of President John Quincy Adams. A lawyer he served in The Massachusetts House of Representatives, The United States House of Representatives, and served as a diplomat to Britain.
3. Edmund Spenser (1552–1599) An English poet. Spenser is controversial due to his genocidal writing. "A View of the Present State of Ireland" called for the destruction of the Irish culture via scorched earth policy.
4. René Descartes. A French philosopher, mathematician, and mercenary, Descartes has been described as the "Founder of Modern Philosophy" and the "Father of Modern Mathematics." He is among the most influential scholars in western history.
5. Chojun Miyagi (1888–1953) Founder of the *Goju Ryu* karate system, Miyagi was a student of Kanryo Higashionna.
6. Kanryo Higashionna (1850–1915) was a native of Naha, Okinawa. He learned martial arts in China and was the instructor of Chojun Miyagi, the founder of *Goju Ryu* karate.
7. *Traditional Karatedo, Performances of Kata 2*. Morio Higaonna. Minato Research and Publishing Co., LTD Tokyo Japan.
8. Jigoro Kano (1860–1938) is the founder of judo. In 1882, Kano founded Kodokan Judo. His parent art was *jiu-jitsu*.
9. Gichin Funakoshi (1868–1957) An Okinawan karate master who formally introduced karate to the Japanese mainland in 1921. He is the founder of Shotokan karate.
10. Morihei Ueshiba10 (1883–1969) was a famous martial artist and founder of *aikido*. *Daito Ryu Aiki-jutsu* was his parent martial art.
11. Napoleon (August 15, 1769–May 5 1821) Was Emperor of France. Napoleon Bonaparte was considered to be a military genius. In the span of a decade, he conquered most of central and western Europe.
12. Buddhist. A practitioner of Buddhism, a philosophy based on the teachings of the Buddha, (566 to 486 BCE), given name Siddhartha Gautama. The Buddhist discipline contains the Noble Eightfold Path.
13. Bodhidharma. A legendary Buddhist monk traditionally believed in Shaolin lore to be the founder of the Ch'an school of Buddhism, known in the West as Zen.
14. *Wutang Lohan Chuan-fa*. Wildish, Paul. *The Book of Ch'i: Harnessing the Healing Force of Energy*. Boston Massachusetts: Tuttle Publishing, 2000
15. Kanryo Higashionna, (see note 6).
16. Kanbun Uechi (1877–1948) was an Okinawan karate instructor. He traveled to China, where he studied a *kung-fu* system called *Pangai-noon*. After returning to Okinawa he taught this system, which was eventually renamed Uechi Ryu.
17. *The Bible*, King James Version
18. Spoonerism n. the transposition of initial or other sounds of words, usually by accident. (1895-1900 after W. A. Spooner (1844–1930), English clergyman noted for such slips).
19. *Random House Dictionary of the English Language*, Second Edition, Unabriged]
20. Chojun Miyagi (1888–1953), (see note 6).
21. *The Way of Healing. Chi Kung, Chinese Exercises for Quieting the Mind and Strengthen the Body*. 1999 Broadway Books, Random House, Inc., New York, NY.
22. Confucius. (551 BC–479 BC) A Chinese philosopher who emphasized personal and morality and justice in his teachings. Confucius' teachings developed into Confucianism.
23. *Isha Upanishad*. Upanishads are scriptural texts of the ancient wisdom of India and are referred to as the end of Vedas. Isha Upanishad is one of the ten ancient Indian religious and mystical writings, which also include the *Kena Upanishad, Katha Upanishad, Prasna Upanishad, Mundaka Upanishad, Chandyoga Upanishad, Brhadarnyaka Upanishad, Samanya Upanishad, Yoga Upanishad, Sakta Upanishad*.
24. Johnson, Steven, "Emotions and the Brain: Fear," *Discover Magazine*, March 2003
25. *The Body Doesn't Lie: A New and Simple Test Measures Impacts Upon Your Life.*, New York, N.Y. , Warner Books, Inc, 1979
26. *The Psychic Side of Sports*, Michael Murphy, Rhea A. White. Addison-Wesley 1978

27. *The Way of Kata,* Kane and Wilder, 2005 YMAA Publication Center
28. Eugen Herrigel. (1885–1955) A German philosophy professor who lived and taught in Tokyo in the 1930s. He introduced Zen to great parts of Europe through his book, *Zen in the Art of Archery*, which described his personal journey to understand Zen Buddhism through the medium of archery.
29. *Zen in the Art of Archery*, Eugen Herrigel 1953 Pantheon Publishing, Inc.
30. Pythagoras. (582 BC–496 BC) was a mathematician and philosopher best known for formulating the Pythagorean Theorem which describes the relationships among the three sides of a right triangle.
31. Tom Brown, Jr. (1950–) Schooled in the Native American ways of tracking, wilderness survival, and awareness, he has authored many books on the subject.
32. In mathematics, the Fibonacci Ratio forms a sequence that starts with 0 and 1, and then produces the next Fibonacci number by adding the two previous Fibonacci numbers. 0+1=1 the next series is 1+1=2, next 1+2=3 resulting in the following series: 1, 1, 2, 3, 5, 8, 13.
33. Leonardo Pisano Fibonacci. (c. 1170–1250), An Italian mathematician best known for the discovery of the Fibonacci numbers and the Fibonacci sequence.
34. The Republic of Kenya, is a country in East Africa.
35. Aesop. (620–560 BC) A slave in Ancient Greece, his famous *Aesop's Fables* are short moral tales typically involving animal characters that illustrate the essential truths about the human experience.
36. Yamada Kenji (1926–), a judo sensei who put together two United States championships in the mid fifties. Trained in Japan, he taught judo for over fifty years in the Seattle, Washington area.
37. Aesop. (620–560 BC), (see note 35).
38. Miyamoto Musashi. (1584–1645) was a famous Japanese swordsman. He is the author of *Go Rin No Sho, The Book of Five Rings.*
39. Sigmund Freud. (May 6, 1856–September 23, 1939) An Austrian psychiatrist he founded the psychoanalytic school of psychology, with the theory that unconscious motive control much behavior.
40. Moore, Keith. *Clinically Oriented Anatomy*, Second Edition. Williams and Wilkins St. Baltimore, Maryland, 1985
41. Henry Ford. (July 30, 1863–April 7, 1947) Founder of the Ford Motor Company. He was one of the first to apply assembly line manufacturing to the mass production of affordable automobiles.
42. Ed Parker. (March 19, 1931–December 15, 1990) Edmund "Kealoha" Parker was an American martial artist; he was the founder of American Kenpo.
43. George S. Patton (1885–1945), A U.S. Army general in World War II. He commanded major armored units in North Africa, Sicily, and the European Theater.
44. Taisen Deshimaru. (1914–1982) was a Japanese Zen Buddhist teacher. He authored many books including *The Zen Way to the Martial Arts.*
45. William Harrison "Jack" Dempsey (1895–1983) was an Irish-American boxer who won the world heavyweight title. His impressive record included 62 wins, 6 losses, 8 draws, 5 no decisions and 1 no contest, with 50 knockouts.
46. Dempsey, Jack. *Championship Fighting: Explosive Punching and Aggressive Defense.* New York, Prentice-Hall, Inc. 1950
47. John Clarke. (1609–1676) A medical doctor, Minister of the Baptist order and co-founder of the Rhode Island colony.
48. Arthur C. Clarke. (December 16, 1917–) A British author and inventor, he is most famous for his science-fiction novel *2001: A Space Odyssey* which was made into a movie by the same title.
49. Lou Holtz. (January 6, 1937–) One of the most prominent National Collegiate Athletic Association (NCAA College) football head coaches of his time.
50. Josh Billings. (April 12, 1818–October 14, 1885).The pen name of humorist Henry Wheeler Shaw, he toured giving lectures of his writings.
51. Kareem Abdul-Jabbar (1947–), an African American former professional basketball player who is considered one of the greatest ever to play the game. He is retired and now an author and part-time actor.
52. Ancient Greek philosopher (384 BC–322 BC), student of Plato and instructor to Alexander the Great, Aristotle is considered among the most influential philosophers in Western thought.

53. Doil D. Montgomery, Jennie Robb, Kimberly V. Dwyer, and Samuel T. Gontkovsky, *Single Channel QEEG Amplitudes in a Bright, Normal Young Adult Sample.* Center for Psychological Studies, Nova Southeastern University, Fort Lauderdale, Florida, 1995, 1996

54. Deepak Chopra, M.D., (1947–) is a medical doctor and writer. He specializes in integrative and Ayurvedic medicine.

55. Real name, Samuel Langhorne Clemens (November 30, 1835–April 21, 1910), was a famous and writer lecturer and humorist.

56. *Sir Francis Bacon.* (January 22, 1561–April 9, 1626) Best known as a philosophical advocate and defender of the scientific revolution, he popularized an inductive methodology for scientific inquiry.

57. Newton's First Law of Motion: I. Every object in a state of uniform motion tends to remain in that state of motion unless an external force is applied to it.

58. Maya Angelou. (April 4, 1928–) Author and poet who has long been a voice in the civil rights movement America.

59 Derek Bok (March 22, 1930–) is an American lawyer, educator and former President of Harvard University.

Glossary

aikido

Created by Morihei Ueshiba, *aikido* incorporates techniques, of throws, joint locks, pins, and strikes using principles of energy and motion to redirect, neutralize and control attackers.

Allopathic medicine

Conventional medicine as practiced in Europe and the United States since the 19th century; sometimes referred to as Western Medicine.

Ayurvedic medicine

A system of medicine, more than 2,000 years old, it is based on a holistic approach to health and illness rooted in Vedic culture.

benshoku dachi

A karate stance where one leg is placed behind the other in a twisting fashion reminiscent of entwined grape vines.

bo

A Japanese word for staff, it is a long wooden pole used as a tool or weapon.

chishi

A stone lever weight used by some karate systems to build strength.

chudan uke

A chest block in the Japanese language

chudan tsuki

A chest punch in the Japanese language

gedan uke

A low block in the Japanese language

hara

In Japanese tradition, the *hara* is regard as the seat of a person's spiritual energy, located below the navel. The concept of the *hara* is used in Japanese meditation and martial arts theory.

Henan Province   A province of the People's Republic of China located in the central part of the country.

Hetero-lateral Neurological Cross Crawl

A repetitive series of marching techniques used in kinesiology to stimulate the brain.

jiu-jitsu

Jiu-jitsu (also *jujitsu*, *ju jitsu*, *ju jutsu*, or *jiu jitsu*), which translates to "yielding or compliant art" is a Japanese martial art, the basic methods of attack which include striking, punching, kicking, throwing, pinning, strangling, and joint-locking.

judo

Literally "gentle way,' judo is a martial art, a sport and a philosophy. Developed from *jiu-jitsu*, and founded by Dr. Jigoro Kano, its basic methods of attack include, throwing, pinning, strangling, and arm-locking.

karate

Translated as "the way of the empty hand," it is a martial art from Okinawa that is a fusion of native Okinawan fighting methods and Northern and Southern Chinese martial arts.

kata

A pattern of movements containing a series of logical and practical offensive and defensive techniques.

ki

The Japanese word for life energy, or life force.

koshi

"Hip" in Japanese, as in waist, or waistline.

kua

Chinese for fist or hand.

kung fu

A well-known Chinese term used in the West to designate Chinese martial arts. Originally, it meant to have skills in any endeavor.

kuzushi

To break in balance or else set up the opponent for a strike or throw.

makiwara

A striking implement unique to karate, the *makiwara* usually consists of a post anchored in the ground with a padded striking surface.

morote kamae

Japanese for "two-handed preparedness," in karate it refers to a standing position in which both arms are held in chest blocks.

nukite

Japanese for finger strike.

obi

Japanese for belt

Okinawa

Japan's southernmost prefecture, Okinawa consists of hundreds of islands known as The Ryukyu Islands and is considered the birthplace of karate.

pneuma

Greek for "breath."

prana

Hindu in origin, *prana* is the infinite matter of which energy is born.

Ryukyu archipelago

An island chain stretching southwestward from the island of Kyushu in Japan. The Ryukyu islands, in particular Okinawa, are considered the birthplace of karate.

sambo

A modern martial art, system developed in the Soviet Union. The word *sambo* is an abbreviation of *SAMozashchita Bez Oruzhiya* meaning "self defense without a weapon" in the Russian language.

sanchin

Three battles or difficulties emanating from mind, body, and spirit.

sanchin dachi

The Three Battles stance. *Dachi* means stance in Japanese.

sanchin kata

The moving pattern of Three Battles.

seiken

Japanese for front fist, or fore fist.

shaolin

A name meaning "young forest" or "small forest," Shaolin is a method of *kung fu* based on eight postures and five animal forms: dragon, snake, tiger, crane, and leopard.

Shaolin Temple

A group of Chinese Buddhist monasteries famed for their long association with martial arts, they are also the best-known Buddhist monasteries in the West.

shime

A form of testing of *sanchin kata* involving striking the performer with open and closed fists.

ski

A physical or mental opening that allows an opponent a gap in which to gain advantage.

Tai Chi Chuan-fa

Commonly known as *T'ai Chi* and translated as "supreme ultimate fist," it is a Chinese martial art known for its slow motion routines.

Taoist

Of or relating to the philosophical system called Taoism, an English translation of the Chinese term *Daojiao*, which means "the way."

triangulation

The process of finding a distance to a point by calculating the length of one side of a triangle, given measurements of angles and sides of the triangle formed by that point and two other reference points.

Uechi Ryu

A style of Okinawan karate originated by Kanbun Uechi.

zanshin

Japanese for "follow through" as in archery or technique.

Bibliography

Chia, Mantak. *Iron Shirt Chi Kung I: Once a Martial Art, Now the Practice that Strengthens the Internal Organs, Roots Oneself Solidly, and Unifies Physical, Mental and Spiritual Health*. Huntington New York: Healing Tao Books, 1986.

Chia, Mantak. *Chi Self-Massage, The Taoist Way of Rejuvenation*. Huntington, New York: Healing Tao Books, 1986.

Cho, Alexander, L. *Five Ancestor Fist Kung-Fu: The Way of Ngo Cho Kun*. North Clarendon, Vermont: Charles E. Tuttle Company, Inc., 1983, 1996.

Diamond, John, MD. *Your Body Doesn't Lie: A New Simple Test Measures Impacts Upon Your Life Energy*. New York: Warner Books, Inc., 1979.

Gendlin, Eugene, T. Ph.D. *Focusing*. New York: Bantam Books New Age Books. 1979, 1981.

Higaonna, Morio. *Okinawan Goju Ryu: Traditional Karatedo, Performances of Kata #2*. Tokyo, Japan: Minato Research and Publications, 1986.

Johnson, Don. *The Protean Body: A Rolfer's View of Human Flexibility*. New York: Harper Colophon Books, 1977.

Johnson, Jerry, Alan. *The Essence of Internal Martial Arts: Energy Theory and Cultivation*. Pacific Grove, California: Ching Lien Healing Center, 1994.

Johnson, Jerry, Alan. The Essence of Internal Martial Arts: Esoteric Fighting techniques and Healing Methods. Pacific Grove, California: Ching Lien Healing Center, 1994.

Johnson, Steven. "Emotions and the Brain: Fear." *Discover Magazine*. March 2003.

Kane, Lawrence, A. and Wilder, Kris. *The Way of Kata: A Comprehensive Guide to Deciphering Martial Applications*. Boston: YMAA Publication Center, 2005.

Kotani, Sumiyuki, Osawa, Yoshimi, and Hirose, Yuichi. *Kata of Kodokan Judo* Revised. Kobe, Japan: Koyano Bussan Kaisha, Ltd., 1968.

Lee, Douglas. *Tai Chi Chuan: The Philosophy of Yin and Yang and its Application*. Burbank, California: Ohara Publications, 1976.

Montaique, Erle and Simpson Wally. *The Encyclopedia of Dim-Mak: The Meridians*. Boulder, Colorado: Paladin Press, 1997.

Moore, Keith, L. *Clinically Oriented Anatomy*. Second Edition. Baltimore: Williams & Wilkins, 1985.

Murphy, Michael and White, Rhea, A. *The Psychic Side of Sports: Extraordinary Stories from the Spiritual Underground of Sports*. Reading, Massachusetts: Addison-Wesley Publishing Company, 1978.

Toguchi, Seikichi. *Okinawan Goju-Ryu: Fundamentals of Shorei-Kan Karate*. Burbank California: Ohara Publications, 1976.

Index

abdomen 91-93
adrenal cortex 8-9
adrenaline 8-9
adrenals 8-9
adrenocorticotropin (ACTH) 8-9
aikido xxii-xxiiix
Allen, Marcus 104-105
allopathic medicine xix
alpha state 103-107
alpha waves 12-13, 103-105
amygdala's 8-9
anchoring 99-100
architecture 79, 92-94, 100, 133
Aristotle 103
arm 59-60, 69
awareness 105
awareness, zanshin 13-14
Ayurvedic medicine xx
back 79
backbone 49
Baguazhang 4
beta state 105-107
beta waves 12-13, 103-105
blood 9
Bodhidharma 1-2
bones 79-80
bow 79
bowing of the neck 55
brain shift 105-107
brain waves 12, 103-105
brain, and language 8
brain, structure 7-9
breastbone 50
breath restriction 141
breathing
    about 91-93, 139, 140
    5:7 ratio 141
    ibuki 139-140
Broca's area 8
bronchioles 8-9
calluses 128-129
calves 110-122
caving the chest 79
cerebral cortex 7-8
cervical vertebra #1 (C1) 55-56
cervical vertebra #7 (C7) 53

cervical vertebrae 49
chamber position 38
chambered fist 69
changes in sanchin kata forms 3-4
chest punch 62-63
chin 54
chishi, about 131-132
Cho, Alexander L. 4
chudan tsuki 62-63
coccyx 49, 51-53
cocoon of concentration 12-13
Colossus of Rhodes 80-81
compression, arm 70
conditioning 4
controlling the brain 10-11
corpus callosum 7, 9
creative state 104-106
crescent step 43
Cross Crawl 11-12
curvature 49-51
delta waves 12-13, 103-105
deltoid muscle 59-60
Dempsey, Jack 72-75
Descartes, René xix
diaphragm 50-51
distance, judging 38
elbow 64-66
emulation 5
energetic roots 99
esophagus 142
eyes 38
feet xx-xxi, 21-22, 24, 100, 110-123
feet, rotating 24-26
feet, testing stance 27-29
Fibonacci Ratio 16-18, 29-31, 72
fight or flight situation 9
fists 61-63, 67-68, 110
flinch reaction 41-43
fore fist 67
forehead 110
four points of the compass 93-94
Funakoshi, Gichin xxii-xxiii
functional view 103
glycogen 9
Goju Ryu xxii-xxiii, 3-4
Golden Mean 18-19

growth pattern 16-18
hands 63, 67
hands, deforming 125
happo no kuzushi 107-108
hara 91-92, 140
head 110
Hetero-lateral Neurological Cross Crawl 11-12
Higashionna, Kanryo xxii-xxiii, 3-4, 147-166
hips 33-34
holds 89-91
Hsing-I 4
hypothalamus 8-9
ibuki breathing 139-140, 142
imbalance 64-65
immobilization 87
inhaling 140
Iron Shirt 91-93, 96
Jacklin, Tony 12-13
jiu-jitsu xxii-xxiii
Kano, Jigoro xxii-xxiii
Kenji Yamada 99-100
ki 83
ki energy 83-84
knee 29-31
knee joint 23-24
knuckles 67, 128-129
kua 19-21, 59-60
kuzushi 64-65
language 8
latissimus dorsi 59-60
learning, methodology 5
liver 8-9
locking a joint 87
lumbar vertebrae 49
lungs 8-9, 51, 139-140
makiwara, about 125
makiwara, drills 129-131
marching 10-11
martial arts, and brain waves 13
median nerve 75
medicine xix
meditation 12-13
meditation, alpha state 13
meditation, moving 12, 14-15
mind 103
mind, body, and spirit 7, 12
mind-body separation xix-xx
mind/body connection 103

Miyagi, Chojun xxii-xxiii
morote chudan kumae 107-108
muscle memory 5
muscle, deltoid 59-60
muscle, latissimus dorsi 59-60
muscle, pectoral 59-60
muscles, in sanchin kata xx-xxi
muscles, thighs 31-32
mushin 4-5
neck 55
nervous system 8-9
Newton's First Law of Motion 143-144
Ngo Cho Kun 4
no mind 4-5
nukite 61-63
Okinawa 3-4
open hands 61-63
pain compliance 87
parallax 37-38
parallax shift 38, 39-41
pectoral 59-60
pelvic girdle 35-37, 53
pelvis 50-51
Pharos (Lighthouse) of Alexandria 80-81
pinning a person 87
pituitary gland 8-9
Plato 103
poker chips 92-94
pucker factor 9-10
punch 64-66
Pyramids of Egypt 18, 80-81
repetition 5
rooted stances 21-22
rooting 4, 99-100
rotating fist 61-63
sacral curvature 49-51
sacrum 35-37, 49, 51-53
sam chin 4
sambo 10
sanchin kata,
    breathing 139
    changes in forms xx-xxi, 3-4
    controlling the brain 10-11
    correct posture 35-37
    different versions 4
    gauging distances 39-43
    goals for success 4
    Higashionna version 147-166

learning 5
    slowing down 7
    and spine 50-51
    stepping 43-44, 47-48
    ten minute 107
    testing 107
    turning 143
sanchin, defined 7
seiken 67
Shaolin kung fu 2
Shaolin Temple 2
shime 107
shoulder lifting 69
shoulders 54-55, 57, 59
skeletal architecture 4
ski 41-43
spine 49, 79
spleen 9
squats 28-29
stance 94-96
stances, rooted 21-22
stepping 43, 143
sternum 50-51, 57
strike 95-96
striking 75-77, 79-80
striking arm 69-70, 70-72
striking fist 72
substantial view 103
Tai Chi Chuan 4
Tai Chi Chuan-fa 2-3
Taijiquan 4
tailbone 51-53
technique 107
ten-minute sanchin kata 107
tensho kata 4
thalamus 8
thcta waves 12, 103-105
thighs 31-32, 110
thoracic vertebra #11 (T-11) 53
thoracic vertebrae 49
thyroglobulin 8
thyroid gland 8-9
thyrotropin 8-9
torso 92-94, 110
tracking 15-16
Traditional Chinese Medicine xx
training 105
triangulation 37-38

tsun 19-21
turning 143
twisting fist 72
Uechi, Kanbun 3-4
Ueshiba, Morihei xxii-xxiii
unconsciousness 13-15
vastus lateralis 31-32
vertebrae, straightening spine 53
vertebrae, curvature 49-51
vertebral column 49
vital energy 84
waist 110
walking 10-12, 43
Wernicke's area 8
Western medicine xix
Wutang Lohan Chuan-fa 2-3
Zanshin 13-14, 105
Zhang San Feng 2

About the Author

Kris Wilder is the author of *Lessons from the Dojo Floor*, *The Way of Sanchin Kata* and coauthor of *The Way of Kata*. He started practicing the martial arts at the age of fifteen. Over the years, he has earned black belt rankings in three styles, *Goju-Ryu* karate (4th dan), *Tae Kwon Do* (2nd dan), and *Judo* (1st dan), in which he has competed in senior national and international tournaments.

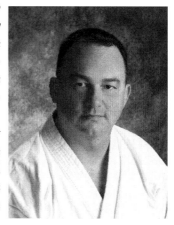

He has had the opportunity to train under many skilled instructors, including Olympic athletes, state champions, national champions, and gifted martial artists who take their lineage directly from the founders of their systems. Kris has trained across the United States and in Okinawa.

A former public affairs and political consultant, Kris' work has ranged from local issues to presidential campaigns. His business client list included several multistate corporations with interests in telecommunications and property development. As a former United States Senate staffer he also worked in the Washington State legislature. He now teaches karate full time. Kris can be reached via e-mail at kwilder@quidnunc.net or visit www.westseatttlekarate.com.

THE WAY TO BLACK BELT

A Comprehensive Guide to Rapid, Rock-Solid Results

by Lawrence A. Kane & Kris Wilder

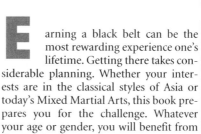

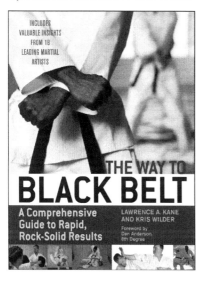

E arning a black belt can be the most rewarding experience one's lifetime. Getting there takes considerable planning. Whether your interests are in the classical styles of Asia or today's Mixed Martial Arts, this book prepares you for the challenge. Whatever your age or gender, you will benefit from the wisdom of master martial artists around the globe who share more than 300 years of personal training experiences. Benefit from their guidance during your development into a first-class black belt.

Featuring…

• Iain Abernethy	• Dan Anderson
• Loren Christensen	• Jeff Cooper
• Wim Demeere	• Aaron Fields
• Rory Miller	• Martina Sprague
• Phillip Starr	• Jeff Stevens …and more.

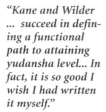

> *"Kane and Wilder ... succeed in defining a functional path to attaining yudansha level... In fact, it is so good I wish I had written it myself."*
>
> – Patrick McCarthy, Hanshi 8th dan

> *"...how much faster I would have advanced... how much further along I'd be today if I'd have read this book... at the beginning of my journey into martial arts ..."*
>
> – Alain Burrese, J.D., former US Army 2nd Infantry Div. Scout Sniper School instructor

> *"... this book... illuminates a path far beyond [its] goal."*
>
> – Christopher Caile, 6th dan black belt, Editor of FightingArts.com.

Packed with actionable information, the authors will teach you how to set goals, find a good instructor, monitor your progress, overcome plateaus, take advantage of every learning opportunity, and work through injuries that come with rigorous martial arts training.

Putting your skills to the test at each developmental stage of your training requires a certain mental 'clarity.' The authors examine what this means, how to find it, and how to make sure that when the time comes you are 100% prepared.

If you are serious about your martial arts training, The Way to Black Belt will arm you with the information you need to swiftly become a highly skilled, well-qualified black belt.

300 pages • 200 photos and illustrations
Code: B0852 • ISBN: 978-1-59439-085-2

 SKILL LEVEL
Ⓘ Ⓘ Ⓘ

Lawrence A. Kane *began martial arts training in 1970. He's co-author of* The Way of Kata, *and the author of* Surviving Armed Assaults. *He's a black belt in Goju Ryu karate, and has studied traditional Asian martial arts, medieval European combat, and modern close-quarters weapons. Lawrence Kane lives and teaches Goju Ryu karate in Seattle, Washington.*

Kris Wilder *began his martial arts training in 1976. He is the co-author of* The Way of Kata, *and the author of* The Way of Sanchin Kata. *He has earned black belts in Taekwondo, Kodokan judo, and Goju Ryu karate. Wilder has trained under world-class martial artists, including Kenji Yamada (back-to-back United States judo grand champion), John Roseberry (founder of Shorei-Shobukan karate), and Hiroo Ito (student of Kori Hisataka, the founder of Shorinji-Ryu Kenkokan karate). Kris Wilder lives and teaches Goju Ryu karate in Seattle, Washington.*

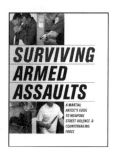

SURVIVING ARMED ASSAULTS—A Martial Artist's Guide to Weapons, Street Violence, and Countervailing Force

Lawrence A. Kane

Fair Fight? Not likely. Least of all from a criminal who is looking to make a quick profit at your expense.

This extensive book teaches proven survival skills that can keep you safe on the street. A multitude of real-life scenarios and case studies analyzing violent encounters will help you to internalize this crucial knowledge. A must for reality self-defense training.

360 pages • 190 photographs
Code: B0711 • ISBN: 978-1-59439-071-1

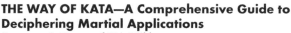 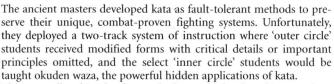

SKILL LEVEL
(I) (II) (III)

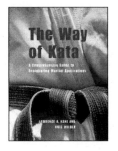

THE WAY OF KATA—A Comprehensive Guide to Deciphering Martial Applications

Lawrence A. Kane and Kris Wilder

The ancient masters developed kata as fault-tolerant methods to preserve their unique, combat-proven fighting systems. Unfortunately, they deployed a two-track system of instruction where 'outer circle' students received modified forms with critical details or important principles omitted, and the select 'inner circle' students would be taught okuden waza, the powerful hidden applications of kata.

This groundbreaking book unveils the methods of teaching you how to analyze your kata, to understand what it is trying to tell you. It also helps you to utilize your fighting techniques more effectively—both in self-defense and in tournament applications. Offers fifteen general principles to identify effective techniques, and twelve discrete rules for deciphering martial applications within your kata.

310 pages • 156 illus.
Code: B0584 • ISBN: 1-59439-058-4

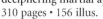

SKILL LEVEL
(I) (II) (III)

BOOKS FROM YMAA

6 HEALING MOVEMENTS	B906
101 REFLECTIONS ON TAI CHI CHUAN	B868
108 INSIGHTS INTO TAI CHI CHUAN—A STRING OF PEARLS	B582
A WOMAN'S QIGONG GUIDE	B833
ADVANCING IN TAE KWON DO	B072X
ANCIENT CHINESE WEAPONS	B671
ANALYSIS OF SHAOLIN CHIN NA 2ND ED.	B0002
THE ART OF HOJO UNDO—POWER TRAINING FORTRADITIONAL KARATE	B1361
ARTHRITIS RELIEF—CHINESE QIGONG FOR HEALING & PREVENTION, 3RD ED.	B0339
BACK PAIN RELIEF—CHINESE QIGONG FOR HEALING & PREVENTION, 2ND ED.	B0258
BAGUAZHANG 2ND ED.	B1132
CARDIO KICKBOXING ELITE	B922
CHIN NA IN GROUND FIGHTING	B663
CHINESE FAST WRESTLING—THE ART OF SAN SHOU KUAI JIAO	B493
CHINESE FITNESS—A MIND/BODY APPROACH	B37X
CHINESE TUI NA MASSAGE	B043
COMPLETE CARDIOKICKBOXING	B809
COMPREHENSIVE APPLICATIONS OF SHAOLIN CHIN NA	B36X
CROCODILE AND THE CRANE	B0876
THE CUTTING SEASON (HARD COVER)	B0821
THE CUTTING SEASON (PAPER BACK)	B1309
DR. WU'S HEAD MASSAGE—ANTI-AGING AND HOLISTIC HEALING THERAPY	B0576
EIGHT SIMPLE QIGONG EXERCISES FOR HEALTH, 2ND ED.	B523
ESSENCE OF SHAOLIN WHITE CRANE	B353
ESSENCE OF TAIJI QIGONG, 2ND ED.	B639
EXPLORING TAI CHI	B424
FIGHTING ARTS	B213
INSIDE TAI CHI	B108
KATA AND THE TRANSMISSION OF KNOWLEDGE	B0266
THE LITTLE BLACK BOOK OF VIOLENCE	B1293
LIUHEBAFA FIVE CHARACTER SECRETS	B728
MARTIAL ARTS ATHLETE	B655
MARTIAL ARTS INSTRUCTION	B024X
MARTIAL WAY AND ITS VIRTUES	B698
MEDITATIONS ON VIOLENCE	B1187
MIND/BODY FITNESS—A MIND / BODY APPROACH	B876
MUGAI RYU—THE CLASSICAL SAMURAI ART OF DRAWING THE SWORD	B183
NATURAL HEALING WITH QIGONG—THERAPEUTIC QIGONG	B0010
NORTHERN SHAOLIN SWORD, 2ND ED.	B85X
OKINAWA'S COMPLETE KARATE SYSTEM—ISSHIN RYU	B914
POWER BODY	B760
PRINCIPLES OF TRADITIONAL CHINESE MEDICINE	B99X
QIGONG FOR HEALTH & MARTIAL ARTS, 2ND ED.	B574
QIGONG FOR LIVING	B116
QIGONG FOR TREATING COMMON AILMENTS	B701
QIGONG MASSAGE—FUND. TECHNIQUES FOR HEALTH AND RELAXATION, 2ND ED.	B0487
QIGONG MEDITATION—EMBRYONIC BREATHING	B736
QIGONG MEDITATION—SMALL CIRCULATION	B0673
QIGONG, THE SECRET OF YOUTH	B841
QUIET TEACHER	B1262
ROOT OF CHINESE QIGONG, 2ND ED.	B507
SHIHAN TE—THE BUNKAI OF KATA	B884
SIMPLE CHINESE MEDICINE	B1248
SUNRISE TAI CHI	B0838
SURVIVING ARMED ASSAULTS	B0711
TAEKWONDO—ANCIENT WISDOM FOR THE MODERN WARRIOR	B930
TAE KWON DO—THE KOREAN MARTIAL ART	B0869
TAEKWONDO—A PATH TO PERSONAL EXCELLENCE	B1286
TAEKWONDO—SPIRIT AND PRACTICE	B221
TAO OF BIOENERGETICS	B289
TAI CHI BOOK	B647
TAI CHI CHUAN—24 & 48 POSTURES	B337
TAI CHI CHUAN MARTIAL APPLICATIONS, 2ND ED.	B442
TAI CHI CONNECTIONS	B0320
TAI CHI DYNAMICS	B1163
TAI CHI SECRETS OF THE ANCIENT MASTERS	B71X
TAI CHI SECRETS OF THE WU & LI STYLES	B981
TAI CHI SECRETS OF THE WU STYLE	B175
TAI CHI SECRETS OF THE YANG STYLE	B094
TAI CHI THEORY & MARTIAL POWER, 2ND ED.	B434
TAI CHI WALKING	B23X
TAIJI CHIN NA	B378
TAIJI SWORD, CLASSICAL YANG STYLE	B744
TAIJIQUAN, CLASSICAL YANG STYLE	B68X
TAIJIQUAN THEORY OF DR. YANG, JWING-MING	B432

more products available from...
YMAA Publication Center, Inc. 楊氏東方文化出版中心
1-800-669-8892 • ymaa@aol.com • www.ymaa.com

BOOKS FROM YMAA *(continued)*